COMPLETE
KRAV MAGA

"Darren Levine is one of a very few people in the world who can critique accomplished Krav Maga instructors, identify pretenders and adapt the Krav Maga system to new circumstances."

—Imi Lichtenfeld, founder of Krav Maga

"Darren Levine's exceptional critical thinking, analytical skills and proficiency in Krav Maga make him one of the best instructors in the world today. This book gives you access to his experience and knowledge."

—Amir Perets, Krav Maga 4th-degree black belt,
former hand-to-hand combat instructor for elite units
in the Israeli Defense Force (IDF)

"An incredibly gifted prosecutor, Darren Levine's mastery of Krav Maga is equally as effective and deadly as his courtroom skills. Without reservation I strongly recommend this book, and the study of Krav Maga under Darren—there is no finer!"

—Scott Reitz, 30-year LAPD/Metro/SWAT officer and
head instructor for International Tactical Training
Seminars (ITTS)

COMPLETE KRAV MAGA

2nd Edition

THE ULTIMATE GUIDE
TO OVER 250 SELF-DEFENSE
AND COMBATIVE TECHNIQUES

DARREN LEVINE and JOHN WHITMAN

Foreword by BAS RUTTEN

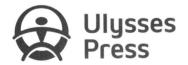

Ulysses Press

In memory of Marni

• • • • •

Published in the United States by
ULYSSES PRESS
P.O. Box 3440
Berkeley, CA 94703
www.ulyssespress.com

ISBN: 978-1-61243-558-9
Library of Congress Control Number 2015952120

Printed in the United States by Bang Printing
10 9 8 7 6 5 4 3

Contributing writer: Ryan Hoover
Acquisitions: Nick Denton-Brown
Managing editor: Claire Chun
Editorial: Caety Klingman
Index: Sayre Van Young
Front cover and interior design: what!design @ whatweb.com
Cover photographs: Andy Mogg
Cover artwork: shield and banner © Maxger/shutterstock.com
Photographs: © Andy Mogg except on pages 3 and 218 courtesy of Krav Maga Wordwide, Inc.; pages
   331–71 © Dominic DiSaia
Models: Tina Angelotti, Jarrett Arthur, Otis Berry, Kelly Ann Campbell, Pawel Cichowlas, Kirian Fitzgibbons,
   Jeff Fredericksen, Ryan Hoover, Christopher Hunt, Jeanine Jackson, Gabriel Khorramian, Darren Levine,
   Kevin Lewis, Kokushi Matsumoto, Eric Powell, Matthew Romond, Jessen San Luis, John Whitman

Distributed by Publishers Group West

Please Note: This book has been written and published strictly for informational purposes, and in no way should be used as a substitute for actual instruction with qualified professionals. The author and publisher are providing you with information in this work so that you can have the knowledge and can choose, at your own risk, to act on that knowledge. The author and publisher also urge all readers to be aware of their health status and to consult health care professionals before beginning any health program.

TABLE OF CONTENTS

FOREWORD
BY BAS RUTTEN

Hey everybody, listen up: This is El Guapo speaking—Bas Rutten, former UFC heavyweight champion, three-time King of Pancrase, and now spokesperson for the International Fight League. If you've ever seen my fights or trained with me in mixed martial arts, you know that I only teach techniques that work in the ring. The same is true for the street—I believe in only doing things that work.

Krav Maga works. I know it does, because the very day I met one of Krav Maga Worldwide's instructors, Amir Perets, he loaded a pellet gun and told me to put the gun to his chest. He said, "If you see me move, you pull the trigger." The next thing I knew, he had the gun in his hand— and he repeated it six more times. It was incredible to observe, and it was simple to do.

Amir later introduced me to Darren Levine, one of the authors of this book. Darren trained in Israel with Imi Lichtenfeld, the creator of Krav Maga. Imi personally asked Darren to be the U.S. chief instructor. If you heard of Krav Maga at all before picking up this book, it was most likely because of the efforts of Darren and the organization he put together.

Darren and I hit it off right away, because he thinks about fighting and self-defense the same way I think about fighting in the ring. Of course, he's not as good-looking as I am, but you can't have everything!

Darren told me a great deal about the system taught by his organization, Krav Maga Worldwide, and I admit I was initially quite impressed. The system is simple and easy to learn. You don't have to be a mixed martial arts champion to perform its techniques. But what I like most about Krav Maga is that it has all the answers. In fact, I gained so much respect for both Darren and Krav Maga that I attended a martial arts trade show with him in 1999. He was the keynote speaker, and once I heard him talk, I became even more impressed. Darren has the ability to explain the Krav Maga system so that it is both easy to understand and obvious.

Darren Levine is one of the best instructors I have ever seen—maybe *the* best—and, believe me, I have seen a lot of them! He specializes in "defense against armed attackers and multiple armed attackers," "hand-to-hand combat without weapons," "street self-defense for civilians," and the list goes on and on. The fact that he also teaches Special Ops troops, FBI, elite counter terrorism units, federal law agencies, and many more, speaks volumes about his qualities. Even professional fighters like me can learn a *lot* from Darren. He's ethical, professional, and responsible. You can tell that I am very impressed with him, can't you?

Krav Maga is a great system, Darren is a great teacher, and you'll find this to be a great book.

Bas Rutten
Thousand Oaks, California
June 2007

In the fall of 2000, a teenage girl named Wendy (her name has been changed to protect her identity) was riding on a bus with her church band. The bus stopped at a mall, and Wendy got out to use the restroom. As is the case in many malls, the public bathroom was located far from regular foot traffic, through a steel door and down a lonely hallway. Wendy walked down this corridor and found the restroom. As she exited the room into the long hallway, a man grabbed her from behind, his huge arms wrapping around her body. Before she could even think, Wendy twisted in place, sending back one elbow and then the other, striking him in the face. Startled, her attacker let go. Wendy spun around and, as blood poured from her attacker's nose, she punched him one more time and then ran.

Wendy wasn't just a member of her church band. She was also a student of Krav Maga.

• • •

This is the story of a Denver Police Department officer. On his own initiative, he appeared at one of Krav Maga Worldwide's Law Enforcement Training courses in Denver to give a testimonial to the officers who were training. What follows is his story, told in his own words:

> In the spring of 2005, I was doing traffic enforcement and pulled over a drunk driver. The guy was totally uncooperative and drunk, cussing, saying he's not going to get out of the car. I opened the driver door and used a twist lock to get the suspect out of the car. As he exited the car, I felt the suspect start to spin on me and saw him making a punching movement towards my head. I had just gone through a Krav Maga edged-weapon instructor course so I blocked what I thought was a punch and used an elbow strike to his head as a counterattack. I heard something metal hit the ground and saw a large folding knife lying next to us. I immediately followed up with knee strikes and the suspect collapsed to the ground. When I took the suspect to jail to book him, we noticed that he had large scars and cut marks across his chest in the shape of X's. I asked him where he got those scars and the suspect said that he had been in a lot of knife fights. When we ran his rap sheet, we found he had been arrested 17 times and most of them for ADW ("assault with a deadly weapon") with a knife. This guy was a knife fighter.
>
> I have a background in Thai boxing, jeet kune do, and mixed martial arts. Although I liked Krav Maga, I thought I would use something else in the field. But Krav Maga came out of me so naturally that I didn't even think about what I was doing and I never saw the knife, only the punch. I am totally sold on KM and you should take the training seriously.

These are just two of the real-life stories and testimonials from people who have saved their lives using Krav Maga as taught by our company, Krav Maga Worldwide. Some are law enforcement officers, some are military personnel, and others are civilians. They come from many walks of life and represent all levels of experience and physical fitness. These people share just one thing in common: They all train in Krav Maga.

WHAT IS KRAV MAGA?

Krav Maga (pronounced KRAHV muh-GAH, which means "contact combat" in Hebrew) is a simple, aggressive, easy-to-learn and easy-to-remember system of self-defense. Krav Maga training focuses on principles rather than techniques because no two attacks are ever the same. No two people are the same. And, in fact, the same person confronted with a certain threat will react differently one day compared to another day.

The essence of Krav Maga can be understood by defining some of these principles. Among the principles that make up the Krav Maga system are the following:

- Techniques should be movements based on natural instincts.
- Techniques must address the immediate danger.
- Techniques must defend and counterattack simultaneously.
- One defense must work against a variety of attacks.
- The system should be integrated so that movements learned in one area of the system complement, rather than contradict, movements in another area.
- Techniques must be accessible to the average person, not just athletes.
- Techniques must work from a position of disadvantage.
- Training must include the stress experienced in real attacks.

These principles guide our training and our assessment of techniques. When we find a weakness in a technique, or when a variation is considered, we ask questions based on these guidelines. For instance, if an instructor suggests a change in a technique, we don't test it with our best athletes, we go to some of our least-athletic students and see if they can perform the new technique (principle: techniques must be accessible to the average person).

When judging a defensive technique, we measure its effectiveness by how well it works if we are late (principle: techniques must work from a position of disadvantage). If the technique only works when we are early or prepared, then we look for something better.

We were working on some defensive tactics with law enforcement officers from the Azusa, California, police department, matching Krav Maga's techniques with some of their already-established team tactics during room entries. Our favorite moment in the training program was when we found a problem matching one of our weapon-retention techniques to their officer's position during the entry. As we explored a solution, one of the officers suggested a particular type of footwork that was different than anything else we had shown. The other officer immediately replied, "No, that would be the only time we'd have our guys step that way. Either he'd never do it because it was so different, or doing it would mess up the rest of his training." That officer understood Krav Maga.

KRAV MAGA IS NOT A MARTIAL ART

One thing to keep in mind as you read this book is that Krav Maga is not a traditional martial art—in fact, we don't use the term "martial art" at all. Traditional martial arts tend to be rigid, dogmatic, and focused on maintaining traditions handed down from past masters. In addition, depending on the art, there is an emphasis on elegance of movement and minutia of detail. Krav Maga tries to avoid all these things. The majority of martial arts systems also tend to become trapped in a sports-oriented mentality, establishing rules that limit the fighters. Even mixed martial arts fighters, many of whom are our friends and whom we respect immensely, fight in a controlled environment with restrictions on what they can and cannot do.

Some very effective systems can also fall into the sports-oriented trap. For instance, Brazilian jiu jitsu (BJJ) is an extremely effective system. Anyone interested in becoming highly proficient at groundfighting should absolutely spend time training with one of the many Brazilian jiu jitsu instructors available around the world. However, many schools teach BJJ as a sport: no striking, no biting, no eye-gouging, and no emphasis on getting up and away from danger. The truth is, these limitations are necessary in order for beginners to practice the techniques (it's hard to practice a triangle choke if your partner is biting your thigh), but if you never add the other elements of a street fight, you are training in a sport, not in self-defense.

This is where Krav Maga is different. We certainly create training drills and training methods that limit student options...but we constantly (our students might say obsessively!) remind them that they should not be fighting by the rules. For example, they should look to disengage and run away, or find an object to use as a weapon. We have no interest in proving to ourselves or the attacker that we can do a particular technique. Our only interest is in going home safely.

Krav Maga is heavy on the "martial" and not much into the "art." We aren't always pretty, but we get the job done. We prefer to describe Krav Maga as a "defensive tactics system"—a tactical and logically sound approach to dealing with violent confrontations.

THE ROOTS OF THE SYSTEM

The founder of Krav Maga, Imi Lichtenfeld, was born in 1910 in Hungary, but grew up in Bratislava, Czechoslovakia. A natural athlete, Imi won the Slovakian Youth Wrestling Championship in 1928, and a year later won the adult championship in the welterweight division. That same year, he won both the national boxing championship and an international gymnastics championship. For the next decade, he earned a place as one of the premier wrestlers in Europe. However, Imi's greatest influence was his father, Samuel, a police officer and self-defense instructor. Samuel started as a circus acrobat and wrestler, but later entered the police department and served for 30 years as chief detective inspector. He became well-known for his impressive arrest record, particularly his capture of dangerous criminals.

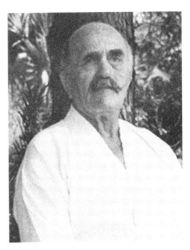

Imi Lichtenfeld, the founder of Krav Maga.

When not on the trail of violent felons, Samuel taught self-defense techniques at Hercules, Bratislava's first gym, which he owned. In training, Samuel constantly emphasized the need for proper moral conduct in dealing with the public and with suspects.

In the 1930s, Imi honed his fighting skills in the streets of Bratislava, protecting himself and other Jews from local fascist thugs. He took part in numerous fights to prevent anti-Semitic mobs from terrorizing the Jewish community in the city. These fights sharpened Imi's awareness of the difference between sport and street fighting. It was at this time that the seeds of Krav Maga were planted in his mind.

By the late 1930s, Adolph Hitler's Nazi Germany had turned Europe into a battlefield and made it a perilous place for Jews. Imi's fights to protect his family and neighbors from anti-Semitism rapidly made him unpopular with the local authorities, and he was forced to leave in 1940.

After several years of travel, he arrived in Israel, which was then called Palestine. He joined the Haganah, a paramilitary organization fighting for Jewish independence. During this time he taught other soldiers basic hand-to-hand fighting skills, and his reputation grew.

In 1948, the State of Israel was born. The fledgling Israeli government asked Imi to develop an effective fighting system, which later became codified as the Krav Maga system. The Haganah was eventually incorporated into the Israeli Defense Force (IDF), and Imi became the military school's chief instructor for physical training and Krav Maga.

This history of Imi and Israel is important for anyone interested in understanding the nature of Krav Maga training. From the moment it was born, the State of Israel was at war with its neighbors. Israel needed to field an army immediately, sending soldiers into battle with minimal training and no time for retraining or refresher courses. For this reason, combat techniques had to be easy to learn and easy to remember under stress, even if the soldier had not had training in a significant amount of time. In addition, the IDF was sending into battle soldiers of all ages and abilities, from 18-year-old warriors to 40-year-old farmers. The combat system had to be accessible to a wide variety of soldiers, not just athletes in their prime.

Imi's solution was to base the self-defense portion of his combat techniques on the body's natural instincts. Instead of deciding what he wanted the soldier to do, he started by observing how their bodies reacted under stress, and used those instinctive reactions as the building blocks for his self-defense system. This approach guarantees that the mechanics of the system stay close to the body's natural movements. Just as importantly, the approach reduces reaction time, especially under stress, since the techniques are close to the body's innate response to stress.

Another element Imi added to Krav Maga was aggressiveness. This attitude was also borne out of Israel's predicament following its establishment. War is always bloody and brutal, but throughout history many wars have ended with some sort of agreement: the winner and loser sign a treaty, and the loser often survives in some fashion. The declared goal of Israel's enemies was to wipe it off the face of the earth. For this reason, Israel believed that it could never lose a war: losing meant it would cease to exist. In response, Israel treated every battle, every war, like a fight for survival. This attitude permeated all aspects of its training, including the hand-to-hand combat. Krav Maga reacts aggressively to violent attacks, moving immediately to neutralize the attacker. We also train with a "never quit" spirit because (again looking back to the system's history) the results of quitting can be devastating to us.

KRAV MAGA IN THE UNITED STATES

In the 1960s, with military approval, Imi began teaching Krav Maga to civilians in Israel. In 1981, the Krav Maga Association of Israel and the Ministry of Education held the first International Instructor's Course at Wingate Institute for Physical Education. A generous philanthropist from New York, S. Daniel Abraham, sponsored a delegation of 23 members from various cities in the United States to attend. The course was supervised by Imi, then 71 and retired from his military career, and taught by Krav Maga lead instructors Shike Barak, Eyal Yanilov, and Ruevin Moimon. Darren Levine was selected as one of the delegates because of his martial arts and boxing background, as well as his involvement in the physical education program at Heschel Day School near L.A.

The course was a six-week intensive course that involved over eight hours of training per day, six days per week. The course was exhausting, and by the end only a few people passed. Darren was one of them.

During the course, Imi and Darren became friends, and Imi promised Darren that he would visit him in the United States. True to his word, in the summer of 1982 Imi traveled to Los Angeles and lived with Darren and his family while teaching Darren more about Krav Maga.

Darren tells a story about Imi's visit, a story that he also told while delivering a eulogy at Imi's funeral in 1998.

> *When Imi came to visit me, I had just bought a new sports car and I was really excited to show it to him. I was really proud of that car. But when Imi got in the car, he started shifting and fidgeting around, reaching over his shoulder. He looked unhappy. Finally, I asked him what was wrong. He said, "This car isn't good. The seat belt, it's too far back. I can't reach it with my right hand. I can't reach it with my left hand. I'm a lazy one. It needs to be easy, or people won't wear their seat belt. It's not safe."*
>
> *At the time, I was just disappointed. I wanted him to be impressed with my car. But later I realized that he looked at that seat belt the same way he looked at everything. It had to be simple, effective, or people wouldn't be able to do it. That was Krav Maga.*

Darren's training continued, and in 1984 he received his full instructor's degree from Wingate Institute. That year, Imi gave Darren his own personal black belt. Years later, Imi would award Darren with a Founder's Diploma, one of only two Imi gave before his death. Darren and his colleagues had already formed the Krav Maga Association of America, and the growth of Krav Maga in the United States had begun.

KRAV MAGA FOR LAW ENFORCEMENT

In 1987, Darren and his top students began teaching Krav Maga to law enforcement in the United States. Under Imi's guidance, Darren adapted Krav Maga to the needs of U.S. law enforcement and military personnel. The first agency to adopt Krav Maga into its force training curriculum was the Illinois State Police. When Darren taught them, Imi, then 77, flew out from Israel to attend.

Since that time, Krav Maga's involvement with law enforcement has grown rapidly. Krav Maga Worldwide (our company, which received a master license from the Krav Maga Association of America) now trains over 400 law enforcement agencies at the federal, state, and local levels.

In many ways, law enforcement agencies share the same needs that the Israeli military felt after its birth: limited training time, limited opportunities for retraining, and a wide variety in officer abilities. Krav Maga is the obvious answer for them.

Some individuals, knowing how aggressive Krav Maga can be, raise an eyebrow when they hear that we teach law enforcement officers. After all, law enforcement work is different from military work: war is to kill or be killed, but we demand more restraint from police officers. We agree with this sentiment completely, and we include use-of-force education and escalation/de-escalation drills in all our law enforcement training.

Having said that, we have also discovered an interesting aspect of Krav Maga's aggressive approach. Because we train officers to go from a non-aggressive to aggressive state immediately, they usually neutralize a violent subject very quickly. The more quickly the subject is neutralized, the less of a fight there is. Less fight equals less damage. The result: Agencies often find that use-of-force complaints decrease once they adopt Krav Maga training.

AN APPROACH BASED ON PRINCIPLES

As we discussed earlier, the Krav Maga self-defense system is based on principles. We do have specific techniques, of course, but students should never mistake the technique for the absolute truth. When looking at the techniques in this book, keep this in mind: The technique is the beginning of your understanding of self-defense, not the end. For example, here you see a defense against a bearhug. The defender creates leverage on the attacker's neck by reaching around with her far-side hand, catching his face and his nose, and peeling or rolling his chin off her chest.

This is an excellent technique…but it is only an example of the principle. You can perform a similar technique by using the near-side hand and digging/pushing against the attacker's nose and eyes. Is one technique better than the other? No! In one situation the first may be better, in a second situation the second may give better results. The point is that you must not mistake the technique for the principle. The technique (as shown) is to reach around with your arm…but the principle is to create leverage on the neck.

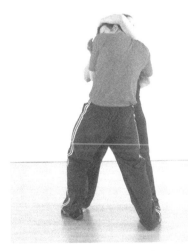 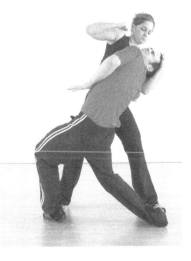 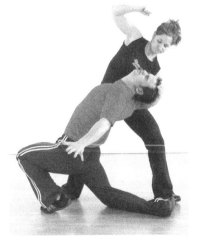

Tina defends against a bearhug.

As instructors, we know that we must start with actual techniques. If we give students abstract principles, they will have nowhere to begin their training. This would be like plucking the strings of a guitar, describing music theory, and then handing the instrument to a new student and asking him to figure out a song for himself. He would feel lost. Instead, we teach him the notes, we help him build simple songs and chords, and soon he understands that the variations of those notes and chords are nearly limitless. So it is with defensive tactics: We start with a basic structure so that information can be delivered effectively. By the end of his training, the student will be able to grasp the theory and make his own music.

FEWER TECHNIQUES THAT SOLVE MORE PROBLEMS

Our approach has always been to find one general movement that deals with as many variations in the attack as possible. It is absolutely impossible to create one unique defense against every possible type of attack. Life just doesn't work that way. If we teach you 300 defenses against 300 attacks, you'll put this book down, go outside, and be assaulted by attack No. 301.

Instead, we try to create one movement that addresses as many variations as possible (using principles as discussed earlier). This yields a simpler, more refined system that is easier to recall under stress. The simpler the system, the more decisive your actions will be because you will not be confused by options.

There is a well-known theory in the study of human movement and reaction known as Hick's Law or the Hick-Hyman Law. Essentially, this law states that the more choices a human being has to a particular stimulus, the longer his overall response time will be. Extended response times are a bad thing in self-defense situations. Therefore, we want to reduce overall response time. There are two ways to do this: a) train more and b) simplify the system.

There is certainly nothing wrong with training more. The more you train, the better you will be. However, Krav Maga is designed for those who cannot train more, and even if you do have time to train, you will still benefit from a refined, efficient system.

Our system is built to reduce your options so that you do not hesitate under stress. When presented with a life-threatening situation, you should react decisively and aggressively, determined to neutralize the threat so that you and your loved ones are safe.

Even if you train enough to overcome the hesitation-due-to-options issue, there is another reason to simplify your choices: stress. Simply put, stress reduces performance. Increased training can reduce the impact of stress, but rarely does that impact fall to zero.

Here is a simple example of the impact stress has on your performance. Imagine that we laid a long piece of wood, a 2x4, on the ground in front of you, then asked you to walk across it without touching the ground. Could you do it? Of course you could!

Next, we lay the same wooden plank across the gap between two tall buildings. Could you walk across it then? Why not? The wooden plank is strong enough to support you. Gravity is always constant, so you are not being pulled down any harder. Why can't you do it?

The answer is simple: stress. The consequences of falling are now much greater. Your heart rate goes up, adrenaline floods your body, you begin to perspire, your muscles tighten. These and other physical and mental responses combine to impair your performance.

Again, training time reduces the impact of stress, but rarely brings it to zero. And since you will only need self-defense techniques when you are under stress, an effective self-defense system seeks to simplify the physical movements and the decision making so that you can perform as well as possible.

EXAMPLES OF STRESS TRAINING

This book delivers a significant amount of information about the techniques and principles of Krav Maga but, by its nature, the book cannot simulate Krav Maga training. Real training involves creative stress drills and applying the techniques and principles under various types of pressure. From our perspective, no technique or response is really learned until it's tested in dynamic situations.

We strongly recommend that you perform stress drills under the supervision of a trained instructor. Krav Maga instructors certified by Krav Maga Worldwide and the Krav Maga Association of America go through an intense training program that includes lectures and discussions on physiology and sports kinesiology. In addition, they attend lectures specifically on safety in training and creating training drills so that the drills they offer are both productive and safe. Ultimately, all the training you do is at your own risk; however, participating in training drills under the supervision of a certified instructor will give you the highest measures of both safety and intensity.

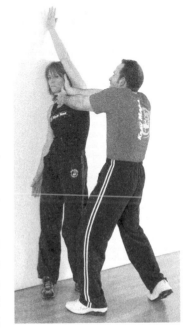

Some training drills can be both simple and effective. Once you've learned defenses from two different types of chokes, simply close your eyes, stand passively, and wait for your partner to attack you with either of those chokes. Once you feel the attack, open your eyes, realize which attack is coming, and react immediately and appropriately. This is the simplest version of a stress drill, and it's quite effective.

More intense versions of these drills include distractions and disturbances. Here is an example involving one defender, three people with large pads, and one attacker. The pad holders begin to hit and push the defender, who can cover himself but cannot attack the pads. He allows himself to be jostled around so that his balance and vision are impaired. At any time, the attacker can grab the defender with any attack (limited to those attacks the defender has learned to deal with). The defender must react immediately. The pad holders then immediately go back to disturbing the defender.

Here's a variation of the drill above, featuring one defender, two people with large pads, and one attacker. Note that this version allows the defender to work on at least one specific strike, and is designed to exhaust the defender and add groundfighting as well: The defender begins to strike one pad with punches, elbows, knees, etc. The other pad holder smacks the defender with his pad, at which point the defender pivots with a hammerfist (you'll learn that in this book) and continues with strikes. This continues. At any point, the attacker closes in, catches the defender from behind, takes him down, and gets on top in a full mount. The defender must reverse the position, get back up, and continue to strike the pads. (Note: To prevent injury, the defender allows the attacker to take him down—a more intense version of the exercise involves the defender attempting to prevent the takedown, but this requires greater skill on the parts of both attacker and defender to avoid injury.) This drill is exhausting!

We have hundreds of such drills that allow our students to learn how to apply the techniques they've learned. It is the only way to truly prepare for a violent encounter on the street.

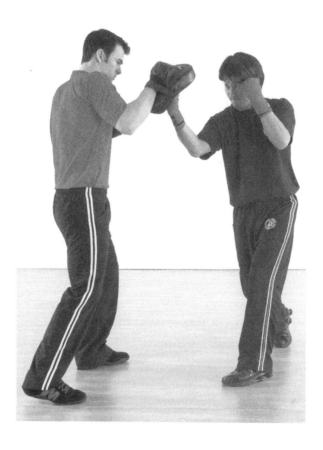

KRAV MAGA PRINCIPLES APPLIED TO BUSINESS AND LIFE

Just to reiterate: Krav Maga isn't a martial art—it's a problem-solving system. Krav Maga is the logical application of a few basic principles to identify a problem and find a solution. In our case, of course, that problem generally involves bad people trying to commit violent acts against us. But there are broader applications for this problem-solving system.

One of the two authors of this book, Darren Levine, is not only the U.S. chief instructor for Krav Maga, he is also a deputy district attorney for Los Angeles County. Darren is a lead prosecutor on an elite unit called Crimes Against Peace Officers Section (C.A.P.O.S.) that prosecutes violent crimes against and murders of police officers. In 2002, Darren was named L.A. County Deputy District Attorney of the Year by the Association of Deputy District Attorneys, and in 2004 he was named Co-Prosecutor of the Year by the National District Attorney's Association. He has prosecuted the worst of the worst: violent criminals who have little or no regard for the rest of society. He has been responsible for the conviction of seven murderers of police officers (one of the highest in the country). And to date he has a 100-percent conviction rate.

Darren attributes a significant part of his success to his Krav Maga training. The logical approach to problem-solving inherent in Krav Maga adapts itself smoothly to other areas of life. One of the most direct applications is to the work environment. Whether you work for the boss or you are the boss, some of Krav Maga's core principles offer lessons you can transfer directly from the mat to the office. Here are a few examples:

Identify the immediate danger. Krav Maga insists on responding to the immediate threat in a practical way. Absorbing this method, you can develop the habit of identifying the actual problem, rather than being distracted by ancillary issues. How many of us have seen a problem at work grow because, instead of dealing with it head on, we or our colleagues have worked around the issue? Krav Maga by its nature eschews this sort of procrastination. By constantly asking ourselves and our students "What is the real danger?" we teach ourselves to look at the overall issue to discover the source.

Operate under stress. Creating a methodology that can handle stress means more than just "sucking it up" or "dealing with it." Addressing stress with nothing more than stress management seminars is like giving bandages to a hemophiliac—you are better off instructing them how not to cut themselves. Krav Maga not only teaches people to function under stress, the system is designed to be usable during stressful situations. In fact, the majority of our techniques work better when the defender is under stress. This approach to problem solving underscores a need in business—you must develop systems whereby stress triggers a streamlining process: Things should move better and faster. Your business model should be like the air foil on a race car—the faster you drive, the more the air foil pushes down on the car, making it go even faster.

Don't trade one danger for another. Krav Maga emphasizes simple reactions that eliminate immediate threats without exposing the defender to additional dangers. Krav Maga's problem-solving process finds methods for reacting efficiently to attacks while improving our position. The tactic translates directly to the business world: When solving a problem, look before you leap—anticipate where you'll end up once you've made the move you're contemplating.

We have a favorite story that illustrates the need for accurate problem solving. A consulting team was hired to do analysis for a Fortune 500 company that wanted to cut spending. One of the areas the consultant team focused on was an annual report the company produced each year in compliance with a government regulation. The company was spending roughly $400,000 per year to generate the report in order to avoid a government fine, and they asked the consultants to find a way to reduce the expense of creating the report. After nearly a month of frustrating, nickel-and-dime effort, one of the consultants finally asked how much the government fine would be. The answer: $10,000. The company was spending $400,000 to create a report in order to avoid a fine of $10,000. The company's initial request for cost saving was a case of mistaken threat assessment. It was an action that removed a danger, but did so by creating an even more expensive one.

Always defend and counterattack simultaneously. You must be able to go from a defensive to an offensive mindset. This doesn't mean you have to be overly aggressive. You don't need to be a warrior to be in business, but you do have to have a warrior's "can do" attitude. Krav Maga training encourages people to attack problems right away, to eliminate immediate dangers because they are life threatening. In business, this attitude prevents procrastination. Recognition of danger leads to an immediate response. Delays in action are alien to Krav Maga training. Responses are appropriate and measured, but they are swift.

Techniques must be accessible to the average person, not just athletes—this is just a fancy way of saying "keep it simple." Whatever systems you implement in your business should be easy to understand. Even if the knowledge or skills required for your business are highly specialized, the systems you employ should be straightforward. The more convoluted they are, the more likely the employees will be to err, especially during stressful situations.

In addition to the principles above, which were mentioned earlier, there are additional training approaches that apply to the working world. Here are a few.

Overcoming Obstacles. In any altercation, you are actually in two fights: one with the opponent and one with yourself. When stressed, exhausted, or in pain, many people feel the desire to shut down.

As discussed, Krav Maga training methods include dozens of drills that teach individuals and groups to overcome obstacles and continue despite fatigue. Our training creates in you the habit of overcoming these obstacles—going over, under, around, or through them—to achieve your stated goal.

Awareness Training. One key element to self-defense is avoiding trouble when you can, which means being on the lookout for potential dangers. However, if you're constantly in fear of threats on the way to your car, you'll never get across the parking lot. Krav Maga teaches simple habits that don't interfere with your normal routine. These habits translate to the workplace in the ability to maintain awareness of potential problems without allowing them to distract you from your goal. This awareness is both physical (enhancing peripheral vision, improving posture, etc.) and mental (creating a state of mind in which the brain takes notice of peculiarities).

Systemic Efficiency. Krav Maga's basic thought process involves simplification and efficiency. We want to create the smallest number of techniques to deal with the largest number of threats. This should be the aim of every CEO in the world. Corporate functions are metaphors for human physiology. In human physiology, the more simultaneous stimuli the brain receives, the slower it is to make a decision. Just so with corporations: The more individuals or departments are involved in a decision, the slower that decision will be. Why create twelve departments when three will do? Krav Maga teaches how to identify waste, and how to retool behaviors and functions so that they cover a wider area with greater efficiency.

Transfer of Knowledge. Krav Maga was not conceived simply as a list of techniques. Because it was created in an atmosphere where time was of the essence, the system developed a process for "transfer of knowledge" so that instructors could deliver a mass of information rapidly and bring people to a high level of proficiency quickly. This approach applies equally well in business, whether during a presentation or in training new hires.

These are only a few examples of the lessons you can take from Krav Maga training into the working world. Again, Krav Maga isn't some secret method for self-improvement. It's a hardcore, practical defensive-tactics system. The more you understand Krav Maga's logical approach to problem solving, the more you'll find yourself applying this effective approach to other areas of your life.

HOW TO USE THIS BOOK

This book is a valuable resource that will absolutely improve your knowledge of Krav Maga and make you safer, but in the end it is only a book. To complete your knowledge, you need to take the information contained here and apply it with a partner, slowly at first and then with increasing speed and aggressiveness. As we noted earlier, techniques are the beginning of your understanding, not the end. Try the techniques as described in this book and use the principles to create variations that are comfortable for your body. Obviously, you will get the greatest benefit from training with a certified instructor. Our certified instructors have the knowledge to teach you the technique itself, and then show you how to apply it under varying degrees of stress. You can find a list of locations certified by Krav Maga Worldwide at www.kravmaga.com.

Along these lines, please remember that a book offers its own limitations. We cannot describe every "what if" situation for every type of attack. If we did, the book would be enormous, expensive, and confusing. In many of the techniques, we describe follow-up counterattacks or movements. These are, for the most part, recommendations rather than requirements. If you feel that a knee is more effective for you than an elbow, throw the knee. Or, better yet, pick up a stick and use that! Our message here is simple: If you take every word in here as gospel, you will gain knowledge, but it will be rigid. That isn't our point. Focus on the principles as much as the specifics.

If you have previous martial arts experience, then we offer you a proverb from Eastern martial arts: In order to fill your tea cup, you must first empty it. In other words, approach these techniques with an open mind. In the end, you will probably incorporate those you like into your own collection of techniques. This is fine with us, but please remember that Krav Maga is an integrated system whose movements are designed to work with each other, not necessarily with movements from a totally different system.

THE ORGANIZATION OF THIS BOOK

We have organized this book to mirror the belt, or level, system we follow in our program. While we don't wear colored belts in our classes, we do use terms such as "yellow belt" and "orange belt" to describe each level of the system because these terms are familiar to people who come from the martial arts world. In our schools, you'll often hear these divisions referred to simply as "Level 1," "Level 2," etc. Below, we've listed the belt color, corresponding level, and the main area of emphasis for each.

BELT	LEVEL	AREA OF EMPHASIS
Yellow	1	basic combatives; choke defenses.
Orange	2	intermediate combatives; bearhugs; introduction to groundfighting; basic fighting skills.
Green	3	intermediate combatives; intermediate groundfighting; intermediate fighting skills.
Blue	4	advanced combatives; gun defenses; stick defenses; advanced fighting skills, advanced groundfighting.
Brown	5	advanced combatives; knife defenses, long gun (rifle) defenses; advanced groundfighting.

The next level after this is Black Belt, which involves additional material such as third-party protection, hostage scenarios, and multiple attackers. Because we can only fit so much into one book, we have elected to stop this book at Brown Belt, or Level 5. You will find, though, that this material covers the most likely attacks you will see on the street.

A Note Regarding Stance: Throughout this book, we have assumed that the defender is either in a passive stance, or in a left-leg forward stance. We prefer a left-leg forward stance for right-handed people. In other words, we have our strong side back. Our reason is simple: Most attackers (especially with a weapon) will attack with their right hand. We want to block with our left and counterattack with our strongest weapon— our right. Once you've mastered these techniques, you should try them from an opposite fighting stance. We require all our black-belt candidates to perform every technique from both stances—but remember, they are testing at a very high level. The average person interested in defending herself will face a right-handed attacker using his right hand most often. If you train for that situation, the odds are you will learn to deal with the most common attacks.

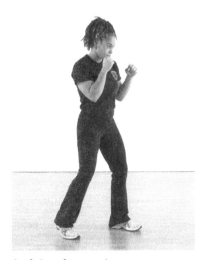

Left-leg forward stance.

SAFETY IN TRAINING

You should absolutely try these techniques with a partner. This knowledge is worth nothing until you've made it your own. However, you must learn to train with a combination of realism and safety. Never be afraid to practice a technique slowly. Keep this phrase in mind: Slow equals smooth and smooth equals fast. Of course, you do want to get to the aggressive, realistic attacks as soon as possible. But trust us, you'll progress faster if you begin slowly and safely.

For this reason, start every technique slowly, with the attacker making a real attack, but at a slow speed and with minimal power. For instance, if you want to train against a choke from the front, your partner should place his hands on your throat and squeeze gently. You should feel pressure so that you can identify the danger, but the choke should not be applied with full power until much later in your training.

As noted earlier, if certified instructors are available in your area, we strongly recommend you take at least a few lessons with them. Not only can they teach you the techniques, they can provide you with some principles for safe training that will bring you to a higher level of proficiency quickly.

The following are additional notes regarding training to defend against weapons. First, NEVER use a real weapon. Various types of training weapons are available, including rubber hand guns, metallic but inert hand guns, and rubber knives.

Handguns: NEVER put your finger in the trigger—our techniques often cause damage to the trigger finger.

Knives: NEVER stab at the eyes, ALWAYS stab at the chest or neck. Even a rubber knife can damage an eye if the defender makes a mistake.

Sticks: Use padded sticks at the beginning of your training. If you decide to graduate to wooden or composite-material batons, train slowly until your technique is correct.

TERMINOLOGY

There are a few words and phrases in this book that might require definition. Many of these phrases are used because we try to avoid terms like "right" and "left." "Right" and "left" become confusing for people fighting in a left-handed stance, and they sometimes stop the mind from being able to switch sides. We've surrendered to common usage, of course, and we DO use "right hand" and "left hand," often for the sake of clarity, but we also use some of the terms below.

Live side: the side of the body from which you can easily launch more attacks. Stand in a fighting stance

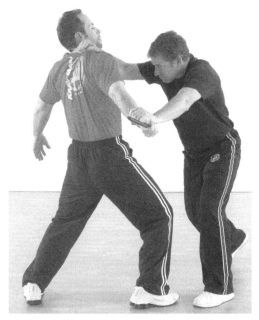

Coauthor John Whitman (right) defends against a knife attack on the attacker's "live side."

with your left foot forward and your hands up: Your right side is your live side.

Dead side: the side of the body from which you cannot easily launch as many attacks. Stand in a fighting stance with your left foot forward and your hands up: Your left side is your dead side.

Inside defense: any redirecting defense in which the defending limb moves inward toward the center of the body.

Outside defense: any redirecting or stopping defense in which the defending limb moves outward from the center of the body.

Inside arm or leg: this term refers to the limb or body part that is closer to the attacker; it can also apply to the "inside hip," "inside foot," etc.

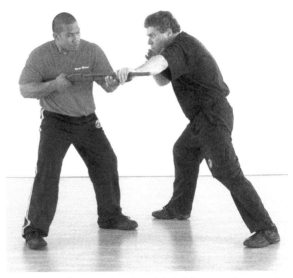

Coauthor Darren Levine (right) bursts forward with his feet to the rifleman's "dead side" to grab the weapon.

Outside arm or leg: this term refers to the limb or body part that is farther away from the attacker; it can also apply to the "outside hip," "outside foot," etc.

Burst: any explosive movement (usually, forward) of the feet. We "burst" in when we do gun defenses, stick defenses, etc.

Guard: a ground position in which one fighter is on his back and the other is on top inside the bottom person's legs. In this case, the top person is in the bottom person's guard.

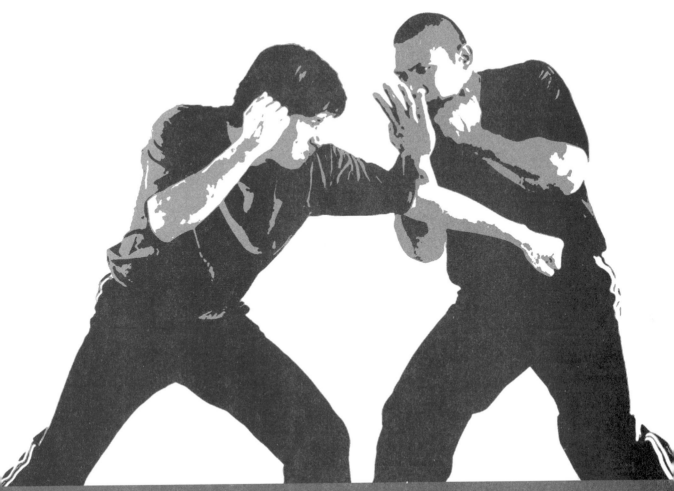

YELLOW
BELT

YELLOW BELT

OVERVIEW

Yellow Belt is the first stage in learning our Krav Maga curriculum. If you attend class at one of Krav Maga Worldwide's certified schools, you will start here at Yellow Belt, or "Level 1." The average training time for this level (assuming at least two training sessions per week) is four months.

The curriculum at this level introduces basic strikes such as straight punches, elbows, front kicks, and knees—the meat and potatoes of a street fight. You'll also learn how to deal with common chokes and headlocks. In addition, the techniques here offer a clear representation of the principles of Krav Maga—ideas such as explosive movements, instinct-based responses, and simultaneous defense-and-counterattack.

Material introduced at this level includes the following:

COMBATIVES

Krav Maga defines "combatives" as the ballistic techniques used both in fighting and in self-defense. The bulk of these techniques involves punches, kicks, elbow strikes, and knees, but Krav Maga never excludes other combative actions such as biting and scratching. Think of combatives as tools to help you in a fight. They are an integral part of self-defense. Even if you're interested in Krav Maga only for self-defense and have no interest in fighting, you must learn basic combatives. While Krav Maga self-defense techniques address the danger, combative techniques are vital in order to eliminate subsequent threats. The combative techniques described here are designed to cause sufficient damage to the attacker in order to remove further threats, while keeping you relatively safe.

Hammerfist punches are made using the meaty part of the fist as a contact point (with the pinky side outermost, toward your opponent). The fist is the head of the hammer, and the forearm is the handle. Good targets for hammerfist punches include the nose, throat, temple, and side of jaw.

Elbow strikes are used when your opponent is very close. Practice elbows in relation to punches by studying the distance continuum: punches are for medium to long range, elbows are for close range. Practice elbow strikes in seven directions, as detailed in this section. Practice solo, facing a mirror. Practice pivoting to strike in any direction.

Kicks give greater reach and are generally more powerful than punches because they are both longer and stronger. Kicks are also sneakier and add more weapons to your arsenal. Krav Maga emphasizes low kicks because they are much more practical for the street. Later in the system we add high kicks to improve our athletic ability, but we always prefer low kicks to the groin or legs. Our motto is: "If you want to kick him in the head, kick him in the groin first; when he falls down, then you can kick him in the head!"

Once you're comfortable with the basic combatives, you should start practicing combinations at various levels and using various strikes. Kick/punch combinations also introduce the idea of a distance continuum. It's important to develop a sense of the most appropriate attack for any given range as that distance changes (in other words, as you move in or out).

DEFENSES AND SELF-DEFENSE

Krav Maga defines "self-defense" in simple terms: The attacker has committed himself to an attack while you are unprepared, forcing you to respond to an immediate threat from a position of disadvantage.

While such defenses as 360° Defense and Inside Defense could be put into the self-defense category when used as reflex reactions against a surprise punch, in general, the self-defense category covers defenses against chokes, bearhugs, headlocks, and other holds. In more advanced phases of training, self-defense will include responses to knife and stick attacks as well as threats with a handgun.

Several main criteria should be used to examine and understand any defense technique in Krav Maga. The technique should:

- Be based on natural instincts/reactions.
- Be simple and usable by people of different strengths and body sizes.
- Work from a position of disadvantage or poor state of readiness.
- Address the immediate danger.
- Include a simultaneous (or nearly simultaneous) counterattack to neutralize further attacks.
- Be comprehensive enough to cover a wide variety of scenarios.

SOFT TECHNIQUES

At times, a less-damaging technique may be the appropriate response to a situation. Examples of such situations include one person simply trying to delay another; a drunken but otherwise harmless acquaintance at a party; and a person holding onto a wrist and unaware of the defender's urgent need to move away.

For these instances, "soft" techniques are designed to remove the defender from any potential danger without harming the other party. These techniques are to be used only if you feel no real threat. If you feel you are in danger, "harder" techniques (especially combatives) should be used.

Wrist releases work off of one basic principle: Move the blade of the wrist through the weakest part of the hold. In other words, take the thinnest angle of the arm out at the point where the other party's thumb meets the fingers.

GROUNDFIGHTING

Krav Maga assumes that, even if the attacker does not try to take you down, you may slip and find yourself down while the attacker is up. This section introduces basic groundfighting positioning and movement. Among the techniques are three basic kicks from the ground: front kick, round kick, and side kick.

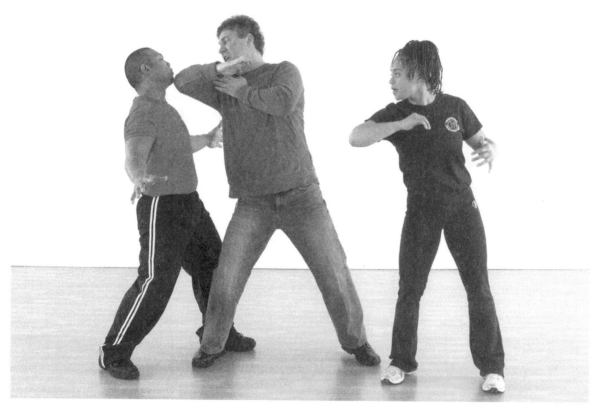

Coauthor Darren Levine demonstrates an elbow strike.

The neutral, or passive, stance is your natural, unprepared position. It is extremely useful for all aspects of training, considering that, on the street, you will most likely need to perform combatives and self-defense techniques without any preparation. Be sure to train from this position at least part of the time when working on combatives, and at all times when practicing self-defense techniques.

THE STANCE: Stand with your feet about hip-width apart (or less), with your arms hanging to the sides.

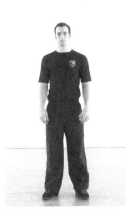

FIGHTING STANCE

Take this stance when preparing for a confrontation. The description below assumes you are right-handed; if you're left-handed, simply substitute "right" for "left."

THE STANCE: Stand with your feet hip-width apart and take a comfortable step forward with your left foot. Keep your weight on the balls (not the heels) of your feet. The toes of both feet should generally point forward, but the forward foot may turn slightly inward for better balance. Keeping your hands relaxed (not in fists), hold them up about chin height and a comfortable distance away from your face. Make sure your elbows are in and fairly close to your body, and your shoulders are relatively squared (not turned sideways) to an opponent.

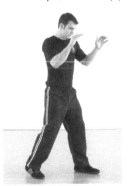

TIPS

If your feet are too narrow, you'll be unstable. If they're too wide, you'll open yourself up for a groin kick.

MOVING IN FIGHTING STANCE

Fundamentals

Even if you're interested only in pure self-defense, you should learn to move quickly and safely while in a fighting stance. The basic principle of movement while in a fighting stance is to start with the forward foot while pushing off with the rear foot, then close the step so you end up in the original stance.

STARTING POSITION: Left-leg-forward fighting stance.

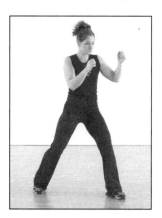

TO ADVANCE: Move your left foot forward while pushing off with your right, then bring your right foot forward to return to a stable fighting stance. Keep your weight evenly over both feet (more on the balls of your feet than on your toes); don't lean forward as you advance.

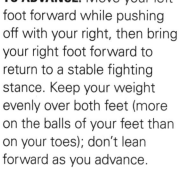

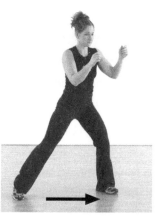

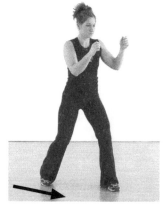

TO GO TO THE RIGHT: Move your right foot out, pushing off with your left, then bring your left foot in so you return to a stable fighting stance.

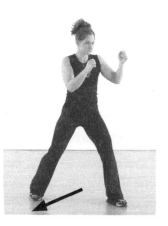

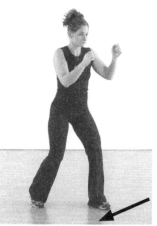

TO GO TO THE LEFT: Move your left foot out, pushing off with your right, then bring your right foot in to return to a stable fighting stance.

TO RETREAT: Move your right foot back, pushing off with your left foot, then bring your left foot back, returning to a stable fighting stance.

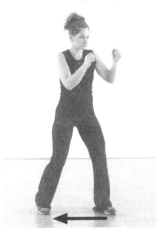

Move with quick, shuffling motions, staying close to the ground. Don't hop! Once you get a feel for the basic movement, practice moving along diagonal lines. These diagonals are what let you advance and retreat while staying out of reach of your opponent's weapons (i.e., not being right in front of them).

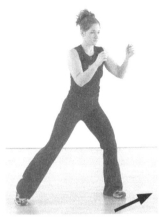

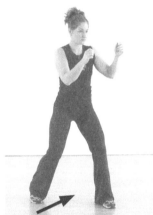

PUNCH MECHANICS

Combatives

A straight punch can be made with the forward hand (usually called a "jab") or the rear hand (a "cross"). The basic principles of the punch are the same for either hand. Although we sometimes use the term "jab" in this book because it is a familiar term to some readers, do not think of your forward-hand punch as a typical "jab." That term implies a quick, less-powerful strike that is useful in sport fighting but not street fighting.

STARTING POSITION: Left-leg-forward fighting stance. Making a fist

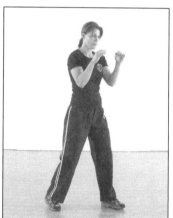

1. Roll your fingers tightly so that there is no space.

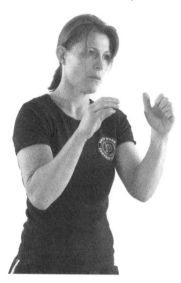

2. Seal your thumb tightly over your fingers near the first knuckle. Do NOT put your thumb inside your fingers!

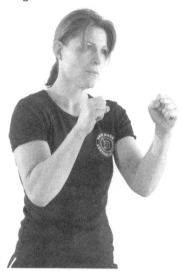

STARTING POSITION: Left-leg-forward fighting stance.

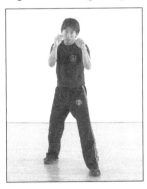

1. Driving with your legs and keeping your elbow down as long as possible, extend your left fist forward. As your hand travels out, rotate your shoulder and hip forward to add power.

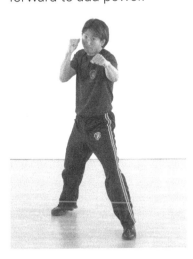

2. Make contact with the first two knuckles of your fist, rotating your fist about 45 degrees to add power. Be sure your wrist is straight. The punch should penetrate the target, not just touch the surface. At the moment of impact, weight should be in the punch.

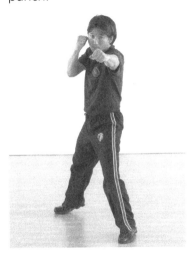

3. Recoil quickly, bringing your hand back to starting position.

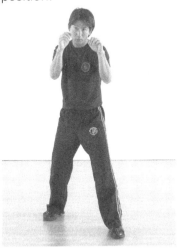

TIPS

Tuck your chin to your chest to protect your jaw.
Roll the shoulder on the punching side up to protect your jaw.
The basic principle of movement while in a fighting stance is to start with the forward foot while pushing off with the rear foot, then close the step so you end up in the original stance.

STARTING POSITION: Left-leg-forward fighting stance.

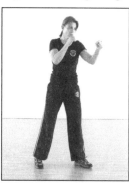

1 Driving with your legs and keeping your elbow down as long as possible, extend your right fist forward. As your hand travels out, rotate your shoulder and hip forward to add power. Pivot your rear foot like you're putting out a cigarette.

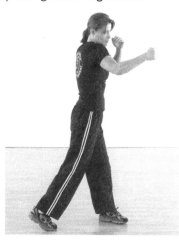

2 Make contact with the first two knuckles of your fist, rotating your fist about 45° to add power. Be sure your wrist is straight. The punch should penetrate the target, not just touch the surface. At the moment of impact, weight should be in the punch.

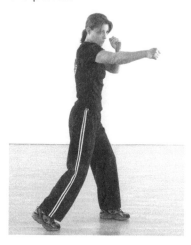

3 Recoil quickly, bringing your hand back to starting position.

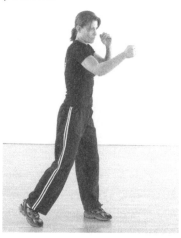

TIPS

Tuck your chin to your chest to protect your jaw. Roll the shoulder on the punching side up to protect your jaw.

You can perform a straight punch using the heel of your palm instead of a fist. The motion of this punch is otherwise the same as a straight punch. This explanation describes a right palm heel strike, but the strike can be done with either hand.

STARTING POSITION: Left-leg-forward fighting stance.

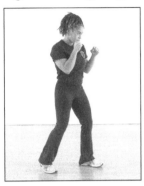

1 Driving with your legs and keeping your elbow down as long as possible, extend your right arm forward. As your hand travels out, rotate your shoulder and hip forward to add power. Pivot on your back foot.

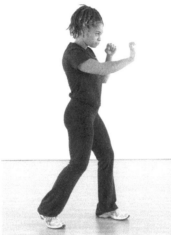

2 As your hand is about to strike the target, flex your wrist backward, open your hand, and curl your fingers slightly, making contact with the hard surface at the base of your hand. Rotate your wrist inward as you strike—this adds extra power and helps protect your wrist. By moving your fingers out of the way, you force the heel of your hand, rather than your fingers, to make contact. If you don't rotate, your wrist may be bent backward on impact, potentially causing a sprain or break.

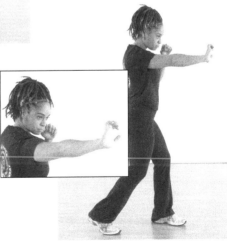

EYE STRIKE

Combatives

This strike to the eyes, another variation of the straight punch, is made with your fingertips.

STARTING POSITION: Left-leg-forward fighting stance.

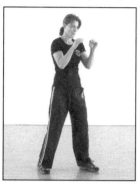

1 Driving with your legs and keeping your elbow down as long as possible, extend your left hand forward. As your hand travels out, rotate your shoulder and hip forward to add power. Pivot on your back foot as if you're crushing out a cigarette.

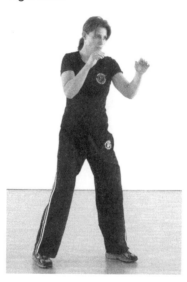

2 As your hand is about to strike the target, press your fingers and thumb together to form a kind of spear blade. Your fingers should be tensed, which gives them strength and usually causes a very slight bend in the knuckles. This helps prevent hyperextension. Stab your fingers forward at a 45-degree angle, rather than straight up and down. This allows your hand to cover the most surface area.

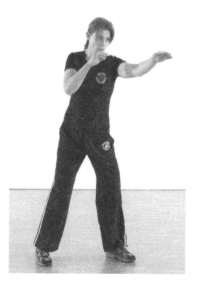

You can make any straight punch while advancing to cover distance. Begin practicing with a forward hand, then try other punches while advancing.

STARTING POSITION: Left-leg-forward fighting stance.

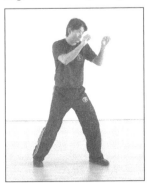

1 Driving with your legs and keeping your elbow down as long as possible, extend your left fist forward. As your hand travels out, rotate your shoulder and hip forward to add power.

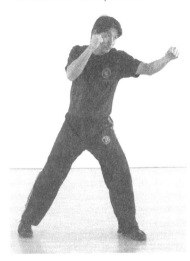

2 Immediately burst in with an advance, pushing off with your right foot and moving forward with your left foot. As the punch lands, close the distance by bringing your right foot forward.

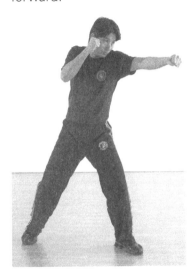

TIPS

In most cases, the advance should be on a slight diagonal to keep you away from your opponent's entire arsenal of counterattacks.

STRAIGHT PUNCH WITH RETREAT

Combatives

A straight punch, particularly a jab, can be given in retreat.

STARTING POSITION: Left-leg-forward fighting stance, facing the attacker.

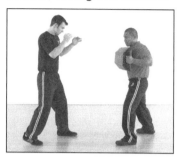

1 The attacker takes a step toward you. Simultaneously send a left punch while moving your right foot back, pushing off with your left foot.

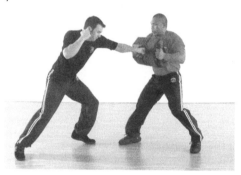

2 As the punch recoils, bring your left foot back to recover into a fighting stance.

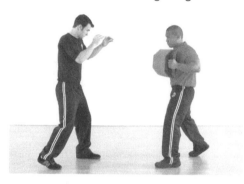

TIPS

The punch may also be performed with a slight duck to avoid an incoming punch.

VARIATION: To make a cross while retreating, you will need to retreat first, plant your feet, and then punch This requires more precise timing than a jab, making it a bit more complex.

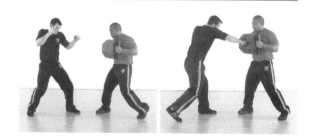

A straight punch can be delivered low—to the midsection or even to the groin. While the basic low punch is the same as a regular straight punch, special considerations require that this punch be practiced separately.

This punch can be made in attack or in defense; see Straight Punch with Advance (page 31) and Straight Punch with Retreat (page 32) for further details.

STARTING POSITION: Left-leg-forward fighting stance.

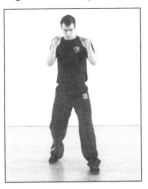

1. Begin a standard straight punch. As you punch, send your fist low while dropping your body by bending at the waist and knees. Do not leave your head up while punching down—this would leave you too exposed. Do not simply drop your body down before sending the punch—this telegraphs the movement.

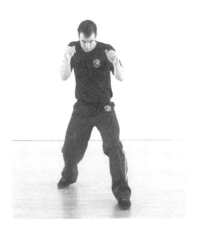

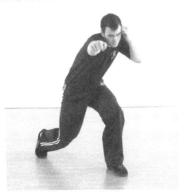

2. Retreat or continue with a further attack. Do not stay down and in front where your opponent can easily punch or knee your head.

TIPS

As with any punch, send your shoulder forward to add weight. This is especially important with a low punch because you need to create a reaction in the opponent that inhibits his ability to counterpunch while your head is low. Practice tucking your chin and bringing your shoulder up to protect your jaw. Practice retreating up and out to avoid counterpunches. Also practice continuing with further attacks.

Combatives

Hammerfist to the side may be practiced from a fighting stance or a passive stance. Because it is often used in reaction to a surprise attack, we generally present the strike from a passive stance first.

STARTING POSITION: Passive stance.

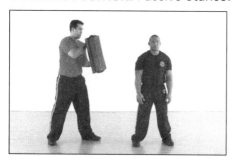

1. Move your left hand sideways and upward, elbow slightly bent. As your hand moves toward its target, rotate your hip and shoulder. Tuck your chin. Your rising arm should cover you as well as strike. Pivot your outside foot and step in toward your target to make sure weight is being transferred into the punch.

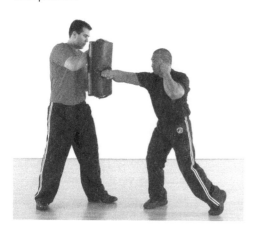

2. On contact, your elbow should still be somewhat bent. The bent elbow should pass your target to help the punch penetrate; it also helps prevent hyperextension of the joint.

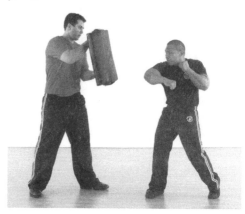

TIPS

Add torque by rotating the fist: At the beginning of the punch, the back of the hand faces the target. Just before contact, rotate the meaty part of your hand out to make contact.

As with all punches, you should recoil after striking.

Hammerfist to the back is essentially the same as hammerfist to the side, but with a greater turn to meet an attack coming from behind. You should practice it to develop the concept that you can strike in a full circle around your body.

STARTING POSITION: Passive stance.

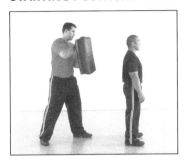

1. Look over your right shoulder. Move your left hand sideways and upward, elbow slightly bent. As your hand moves toward its target, rotate your hip and shoulder. Tuck your chin. Your rising arm should cover you as well as strike. Pivot your outside foot and step in toward your target to make sure weight is being transferred into the punch.

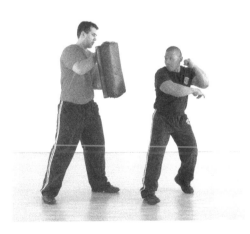

2. On contact, your elbow should still be somewhat bent. The bent elbow should pass your target to help the punch penetrate; it also helps prevent hyperextension of the joint.

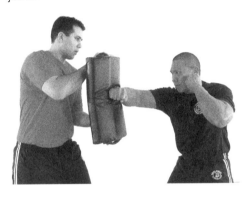

TIPS

Add torque by rotating the fist: At the beginning of the punch, the back of the hand faces the target. Just before contact, rotate the meaty part of your hand out to make contact.

As with all punches, you should recoil after striking.

Combatives

A forward hammerfist is generally a strike to your opponent's face.

STARTING POSITION: Passive stance.

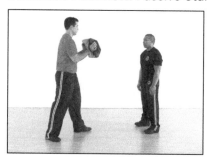

1. Raise your left hand in a small windup—roughly from chin height to about eyebrow height. Don't throw your hand too high above your head—that motion would be too slow and detectable.

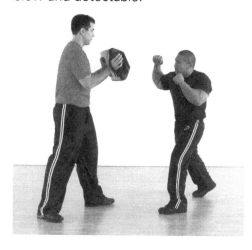

2. As your fist comes down, generate power by rotating your shoulder and hip inward and forward while driving with your legs.

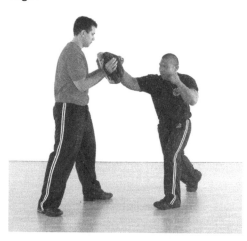

TIPS

Add torque by rotating your fist: As you begin the punch, your palm should face the target. Just before you connect, rotate the meaty part of your hand inward to make contact.

A downward hammerfist will generally be to the back of your opponent's neck, at the base of the skull with your opponent doubled over (for example, after a groin kick). Other targets may be the kidneys (against a low bearhug) or face (during counterattacks against Headlock from the Side or Bearhug with Leverage on the Neck).

STARTING POSITION: Passive stance.

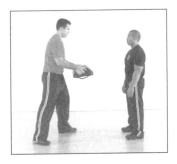

1. Raise your left fist upward in a small windup.

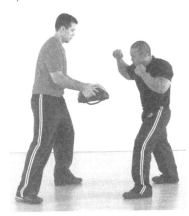

2. As your punch descends, generate power by rotating your hip and shoulder inward and down, and by bending your knees. Do *not* bend at the waist.

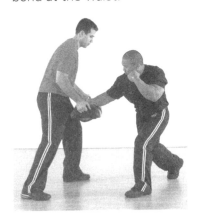

TIPS

Add torque by rotating your fist: As you begin the punch, your palm should face downward to the target. Just before you connect, rotate the meaty part of your hand inward to make contact.

HORIZONTAL HIGH ELBOW STRIKE (ELBOW #1)

Combatives

For training purposes, we start in a modified passive stance. Of course, all elbows can be made from a fighting stance.

STARTING POSITION:
Modified passive stance, with your hands raised up to face height.

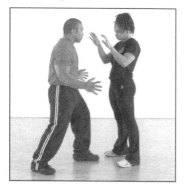

1. Bring your right hand (either in a fist, or open with slightly bent fingers) in to your shoulder, creating a firm bend in your elbow.

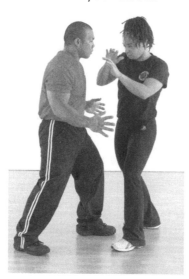

2. Sharply swing your elbow out horizontally in front of you to make contact with your target's face or throat. Strike with the point just below the tip of your elbow, pivoting as you strike to generate more power.

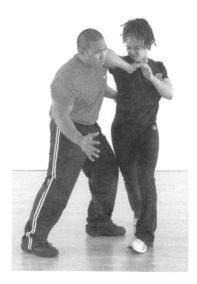

Recoil and return to starting position.

This elbow strike targets an attacker coming from the side.

STARTING POSITION:
Modified passive stance, with your hands raised up to face height.

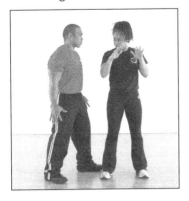

1. Bring your right hand (either in a fist, or open with slightly bent fingers) in to your shoulder, creating a firm bend in your elbow. Raise your elbow up.

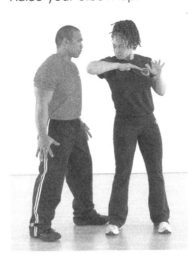

2. Strike to the side, avoiding a "flapping" motion. Lean in as you strike, making contact just above the tip of your elbow. Use your legs for power.

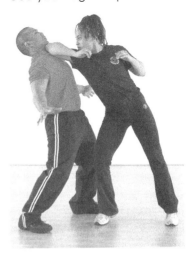

Recoil and return to starting position.

Combatives

STARTING POSITION:
Modified passive stance, with your hands raised up to face height.

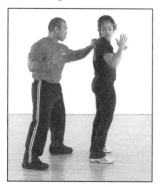

1. Bring your right hand (either in a fist, or open with slightly bent fingers) in to your shoulder, creating a firm bend in your elbow.

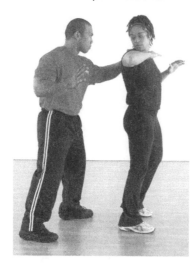

2. Pivot as you punch your elbow horizontally to a target behind you, looking back over your shoulder to see your target (make sure to keep you chin tucked for protection). Strike with the point just above the tip of your elbow.

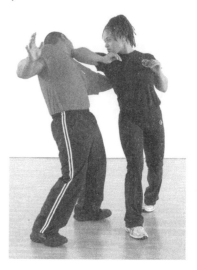

Recoil and return to starting position.

This elbow strike targets an attacker coming from behind.

STARTING POSITION:
Modified passive stance, with your hands raised up to face height.

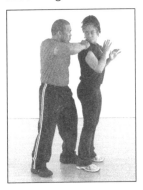

1. Send your elbow straight back to make contact with your target's ribs or stomach. Strike with the point just above the tip of your elbow, pivoting as you strike to generate more power.

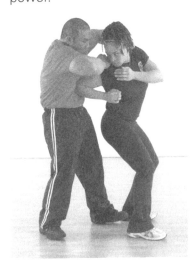

Recoil and return to starting position.

Combatives

This elbow strike targets an attacker coming from behind.

STARTING POSITION:
Modified passive stance, with your hands raised up to face height.

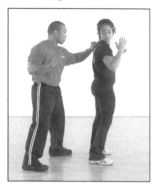

1. Bring your right hand (either in a fist, or open with slightly bent fingers) in to your shoulder, creating a firm bend in your elbow.

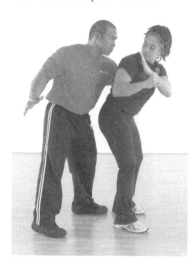

2–3. Punch your elbow backward and upward, tilting your shoulders forward to strike the attacker's throat or face. Strike with the point just above the tip of your elbow.

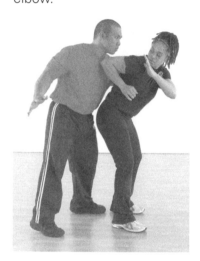

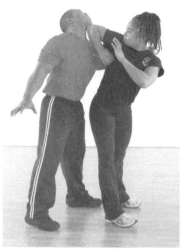

Recoil and return to starting position.

Combatives

STARTING POSITION:
Modified passive stance, with your hands raised up to face height.

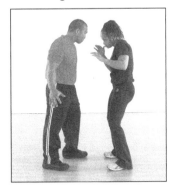

1. Bring your right hand (either in a fist, or open with slightly bent fingers) in to your shoulder, creating a firm bend in your elbow.

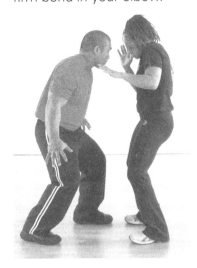

2–3. Swing your elbow up, pivoting your hip and shoulder in and up to generate more power. Strike your target's chin with the point just below the tip of your elbow.

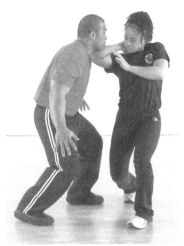

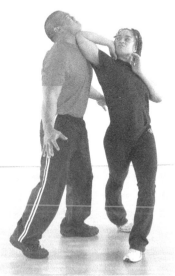

Recoil and return to starting position.

Combatives

This elbow strike is similar to a Downward Hammerfist (page 37). The attacker is poised to attack you from a low angle, or is doubled over (following a groin kick, for example).

STARTING POSITION: Modified passive stance, with your hands raised up to face height.

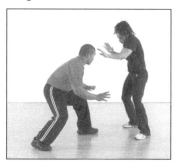

1. Bring your right hand (either in a fist, or open with slightly bent fingers) in to your shoulder, creating a firm bend in your elbow.

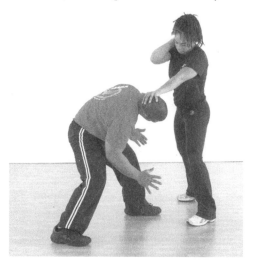

2. Bend your knees and drop your weight down as you swing your elbow down. Strike the back of your opponent's head or neck with the point just above (i.e., toward your shoulder) the tip of your elbow.

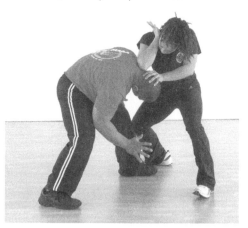

There are two basic front kicks. The first is a regular front kick with the instep or shin (to the groin). The second is to a vertical target using the ball of the foot (page 46). Regular front kick is simpler and more practical in most self-defense situations, so practice it first.

STARTING POSITION: Left-leg-forward fighting stance.

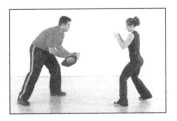

1. Swing your right leg forward, bending your knee.

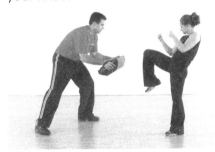

2. As your hip comes forward and upward, snap your foot out, driving through the target. Pivot slightly on your left (base) foot—this opens your hips, which helps extend the kick and add power. Contact the target with your instep, about where you tie your shoelaces.

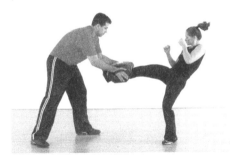

3. Recoil. After making contact, you should be able to either put the kicking foot down in front of you or bring it back into a fighting stance.

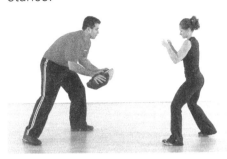

TIPS

When kicking a pad, make sure you look at the center of your partner's chest, not at the pad. This helps you kick through for more penetration, whereas if you just look at the pad, you'll only kick to that point.
Be sure your hands stay up!

VARIATION 1: If you are close to the target, you can connect with your shin as well, which is very powerful.

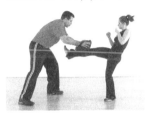

VARIATION 2 (NOT PICTURED): Once you've mastered the basic kick, try kicking with the forward leg, which is less powerful, but faster and sneakier.

FRONT KICK (VERTICAL TARGET)

Combatives

This kick is made to the midsection or chest using the ball of the foot.

STARTING POSITION: Left-leg-forward fighting stance.

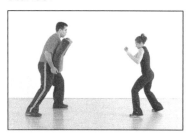

1. Bring your right leg forward with the knee up.

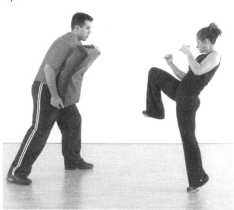

2. Punch the foot, leg, and hip straight out (i.e., not upward, as in the regular front kick). As you kick, curl your toes upward to the top of your shoe, exposing and tightening the ball of your foot. Strike with the ball of your foot.

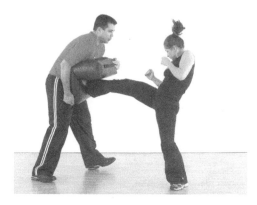

Recoil. You should be able to make a strong kick and then plant your kicking foot to any point, as needed, either in front or recovering back to a fighting stance.

TIPS

Practice kicking the ground with the ball of your foot to help get a feel for the striking surface.

A round kick is, essentially, a front kick that "rolls over" at the last minute. Like the regular front kick, the round kick uses your instep or shin as the striking surface. In a more advanced version, you make contact with the ball of your foot. Round kick can be made to the side of an opponent's knee joint, thigh, ribs, or even head, although we do not emphasize high kicks in Krav Maga.

STARTING POSITION: Left-leg-forward fighting stance.

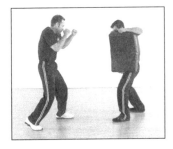

1–2. Swing your right leg forward, bending your knee. Roll your hip over.

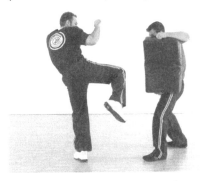

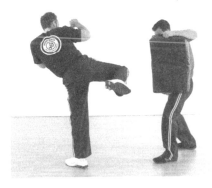

3. Snap out your foot while pivoting quickly on your left foot. Strike with your shin. When you make contact, your knee should still be slightly bent. This lets the motion penetrate the target, and also protects the knee against hyperextension.

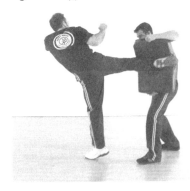

Recoil. You should be able to land forward with control, or bring your foot back into a fighting stance.

TIPS

To deliver the kick with power, be sure your left (base) foot is "deeper" than the target, allowing the kicking leg to drive through. Also, for more power, you may step diagonally and pivot your left foot before sending the kick. Though this adds power, it is more detectable.

VARIATION: It is possible to strike with the top of the foot or ball of the foot.

Combatives

If a front kick is analogous to a straight punch, then knee strikes are analogous to elbow strikes. That is, they are for the close-in fight, and they can be devastating.

STARTING POSITION: Left-leg-forward fighting stance in close proximity to your opponent.

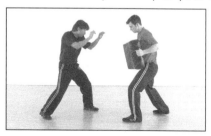

1. Grab your opponent's right arm and shoulder firmly by grabbing handfuls of skin. Push your right forearm against your opponent's neck, keeping your elbow down. This prevents your opponent from dropping down and "shooting in" to grab your legs.

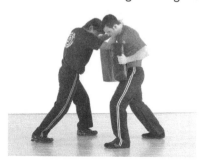

2. Pull your opponent's body forward and/or down while bringing your right knee up sharply, striking the groin, midsection, or face with the point just above your kneecap. Drive your hip forward and up to generate power.

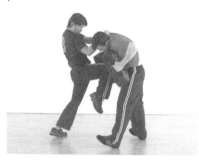

TIPS

If you grab the attacker's left arm and shoulder, strike with your left knee. Be sure your knee is bent sharply.

If your target is the groin, drive your hip forward and pull your opponent's body toward you.

If your target is the midsection or head, pull your opponent's body down while driving your knee upward.

VARIATION: If you place one hand on either side of your opponent's head (a Muay Thai clinch), use either knee for the strike. Grab the attacker by the head with one arm on each side, elbows down and tight. Your hands should be laid one over the other, with your fingers up the back of his head and pushing down to create pressure on his neck, which gives better control. Be sure you squeeze your elbows together to keep your opponent from slipping his head down and out.

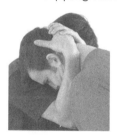

Knee strikes may be applied from different angles. Like a round kick, a round knee starts like the standard strike, relatively straight, and then the hip rolls over. This variation should be practiced after you've mastered the basic knee strike; it's quite effective if your opponent is in front of you but leaving his side open to your attack.

STARTING POSITION: Left-leg-forward fighting stance in close proximity to your opponent.

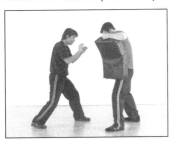

1. Grab your opponent's right arm and shoulder firmly by grabbing handfuls of skin. Push your right forearm against your opponent's neck, keeping your elbow down. This prevents your opponent from dropping down and "shooting in" to grab your legs.

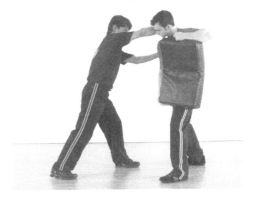

2. Pull your opponent's body forward and/or down while bringing your right knee up; roll your hip over in a motion similar to a round kick so that your knee strikes at a more horizontal angle. This strike is normally delivered to the ribs, stomach, or head. Drive your hip forward and up to generate power.

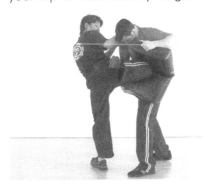

FRONT KICK/HAMMERFIST

Combatives

STARTING POSITION: Left-leg-forward fighting stance.

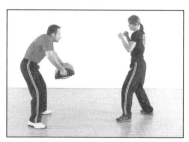

1–2. Deliver a regular front kick to the groin. For this combination, recoil and land with your right (kicking) foot forward and to the outside of your target, not right in front.

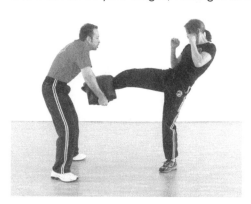

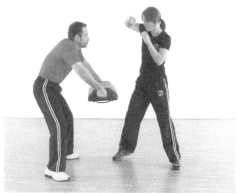

3. As your right foot steps to the ground, use your right hand to deliver a hammerfist to the back of your opponent's neck.

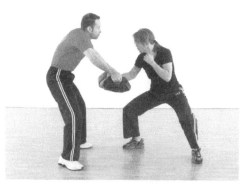

The hammerfist should land almost simultaneously with the foot touching the ground.

STARTING POSITION: Left-leg-forward fighting stance.

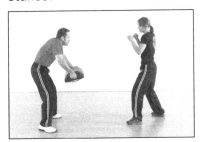

1. Deliver a regular front kick to the groin. Recoil your right (kicking) foot.

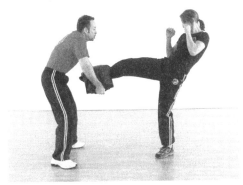

2. As your right foot lands, use your right hand to deliver a straight punch to the face or throat.

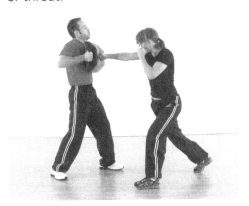

Defenses

This exercise serves as a basic introduction to outside defenses, including defenses against hooks, punches, and knife attacks. 360° Defense is a reflexive exercise based on the body's instinctive reactions. The defense is performed with the fingers extended. This is a relatively instinctive (reflexive) movement, which makes it quick; extending your fingers adds a few inches to the defense.

STARTING POSITION: Neutral (passive) stance, hands up at shoulder/face level. With all these defense positions, make the movement quickly and then recoil.

POSITION 1: With your elbow bent 90°, raise your forearm above and slightly in front of your head to defend against an attack coming straight down.

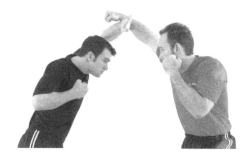

POSITION 2: With your elbow bent 90°, raise your arm at an angle (like the roof of a house—about 30°) to defend against an attack at 45°.

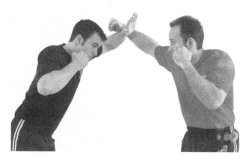

POSITION 3: Starting with your elbow bent 90°, send your forearm out parallel with the floor (with both arms it would look like horizontal goalposts) to defend against an attack coming directly from the side.

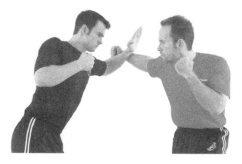

POSITION 4: Bring your elbow (bent 90°) in tight to your body to defend against an upward attack to your ribs. Angle your forearm slightly outward and contract your abs.

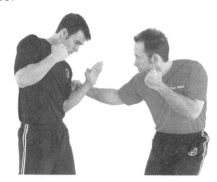

POSITION 5: With your elbow bent 90°, point your fingers down to defend against an upward attack to your ribs. This is the exact opposite of Position #3.

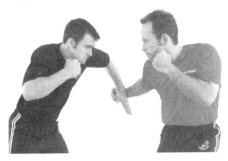

POSITION 6: Starting with your elbow bent 90°, lower your arm at a 30° angle to defend against a rising attack to your body. Be sure to bend at your waist, not at your knees.

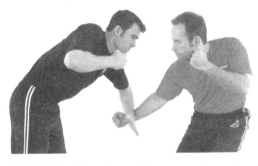

POSITION 7: Starting with your elbow bent 90°, lower your forearm below and slightly in front of your chest to defend against a rising attack to the center of your body. Be sure to bend at your waist, not at your knees.

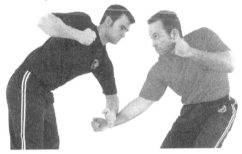

Defend using the blade of your arm. Put weight behind the defense.

Defend from wrist to wrist.

Your partner should attack with very straight arms. While this would be unlikely in a street attack, it makes an excellent training method both for the defense and to develop vision.

Look at the center of your partner's chest and use peripheral vision to see all attacks— if you turn your head to focus on one attack, you will not see an attack coming from the other side.

Attackers should begin slowly, one attack at a time, and increase speed as defending improves.

Defenses

Inside Defense is made against straight punches to the face or throat. Unlike 360° Defense, which is a "stopping" defense, Inside Defenses are "redirecting" defenses. They redirect the attack away from its intended target. Defend with the same-side (mirror) hand. No "cross blocking." For example, if an attacker punches with the left hand, you defend with your right.

STARTING POSITION: Left-leg-forward fighting stance, hands up and slightly less than shoulder-width apart.

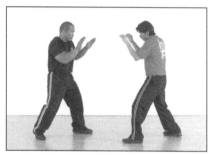

1. As an attacker moves toward you with a straight punch, bring your defending hand forward and inward, pushing against the attacker's arm with the center of your palm. Your palm should slide along the attacker's arm. Move from just inside your shoulder inward toward your line of sight. At the same time, make a small head defense to the outside to give yourself some extra space in case your hand defense didn't succeed.

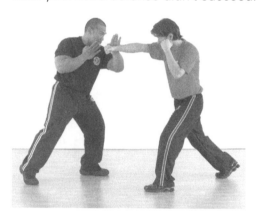

TIPS

Defend with your palm, but if you misread the height of the punch, you can also defend with your wrist or forearm (see Inside Defense against Straight Punch Low, page 55).

INSIDE DEFENSE AGAINST STRAIGHT PUNCH LOW

To defend effectively against a low punch, you must be able to keep your hands up in order to guard against feints or second attacks.

STARTING POSITION: Left-leg-forward fighting stance, hands up and slightly less than shoulder-width apart.

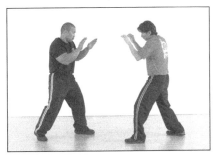

1. As an attacker moves toward you with a low straight punch, bring your elbow across your body in a sweeping motion. As with regular Inside Defense, make this defense with the same-side (mirroring) arm—i.e., defend against a right punch using the left arm. Lead the motion with your elbow; your hand should stay up. Make a body defense by rotating slightly. Against a right punch, rotate right. Against a left punch, rotate left.

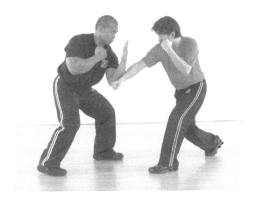

TIPS

Contract your abs to protect your midsection and to lower your upper body slightly so the elbow covers more of the midsection.

Defenses

Once you have mastered basic Inside Defense and 360°, you should begin to defend against the possibility of either attack.

STARTING POSITION: Left-leg-forward fighting stance. From a slight distance, the attacker moves in with a slight advance.

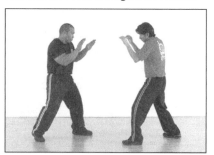

1–6. The attacker delivers one punch at a time, but mixes up 360° and straight-punch attacks. The defender makes the appropriate defense.

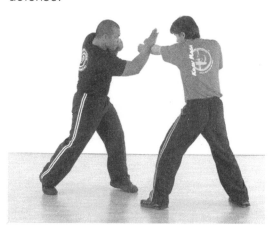

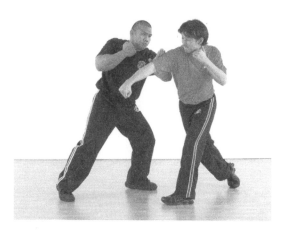

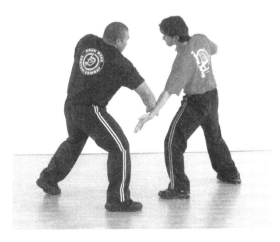

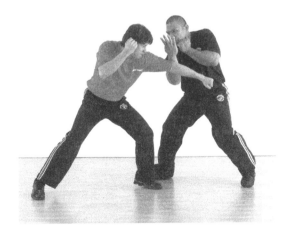

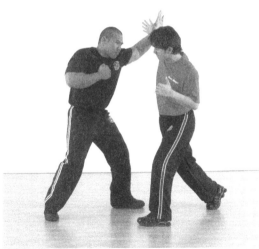

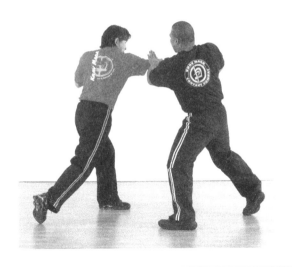

CHOKE FROM THE FRONT (TWO-HANDED PLUCK)

Self-Defense

Choke from the Front is a fairly common attack. It is also a convenient starting point for self-defense training because it underscores many Krav Maga principles. The instinctive reaction to a choke will be to send the hands to the danger—in this case, the throat. This technique turns that reaction into a defense. The pluck is explosive, using speed rather than strength.

STARTING POSITION: Always train on this and other chokes from a passive or neutral stance.

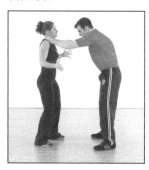

1–2. Using your hands as hooks, with fingers slightly curled and thumbs tight against the hands, bring them up and over your attacker's hands, reach in, and pluck explosively outward, plucking as close to the attacker's thumbs as possible. Tuck your chin to protect your face from an accidental headbutt.

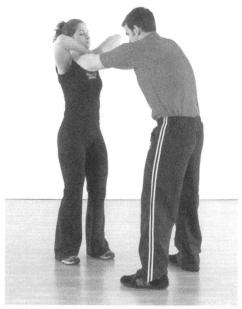

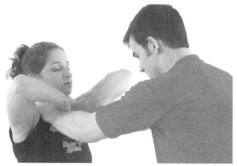

3–4. Trace your shoulder line, then pull down, pinning the attacker's hands to your shoulders. As you pluck, make a simultaneous kick to the groin.

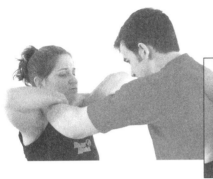
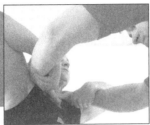

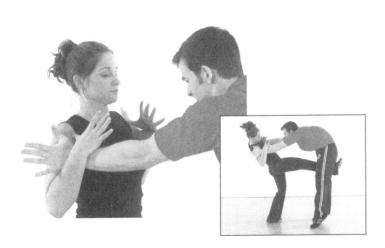

CHOKE FROM THE FRONT (ONE-HANDED PLUCK)

Self-Defense

This variation, while less instinctive than the two-handed pluck, may offer a more performable plucking motion to some people. Also, while it will not stop a headbutt delivered simultaneously with the choke, it will prevent a headbutt given after a short delay.

STARTING POSITION: Passive or neutral stance.

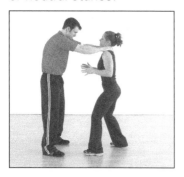

1–2. As the attacker chokes you, reach up with one hand to pluck the attacker's same-side hand.

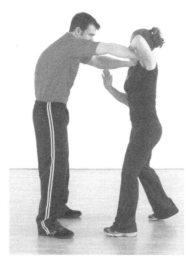

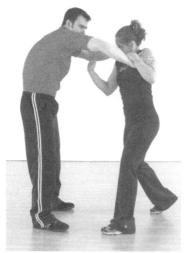

3. At the same time, send your free hand up and under the other arm, delivering a palm strike to the chin or face. (If you're more advanced, deliver an uppercut.)

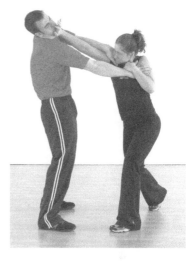

TIPS

Be aware that to deliver a palm strike, you will have to lower the punching-side shoulder to get it below the attacker's hand/arm.
The body rotation made by the combination of pluck and punch should help release pressure from your throat.

STARTING POSITION: Passive stance, with the attacker choking you from behind.

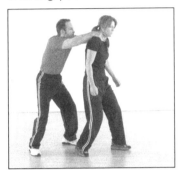

1. Upon feeling the choke, tuck your chin and round your shoulders to expose the attacker's thumbs.

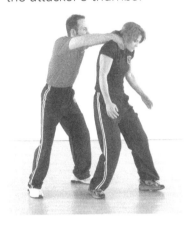

2. Send your hands back as far as possible to gather momentum for the pluck and to ensure that the pluck actually moves the hands.

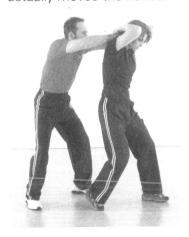

3. Reaching back to the middle of your neck, pluck the attacker's thumbs straight down, as though giving two elbows to your stomach. As you pluck, step diagonally backward, making sure both of your feet move.

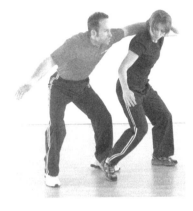

steps 4–7 continued on next page

Self-Defense

continued from previous page

4–5. With your inside hand, strike to the groin and follow with elbows to the stomach or face. This strike should flow naturally from the downward movement of your hand. The outside hand should continue to hold onto the attacker's hand, to keep him close or track his movement until you can make further counters.

6. Turn inside toward the attacker with a hammerfist strike to his face. At this point you can release his hand.

When practicing, break the exercise into two parts. Work on the defense with the groin and elbow strikes first. Then work on the hammerfist, turn, and counter. The initial groin strike can be made with the palm facing the target and the fingers striking up and under for the greatest effect.

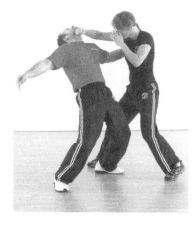

7. Finish with knee strikes or move out to create distance.

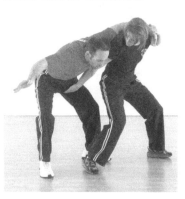

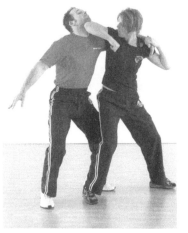

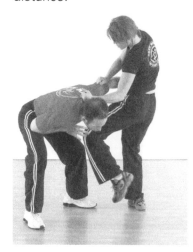

Because Krav Maga attempts to solve various problems with one solution, the same basic principle that worked for Choke from the Front (page 58) and Choke from Behind (page 61) also works with Choke from the Side.

STARTING POSITION: Passive stance as the attacker chokes from the side.

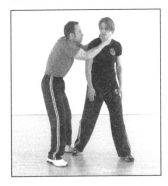

1. Reach your outside hand up and across.

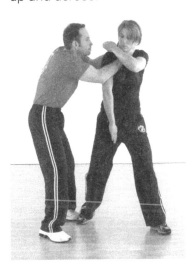

2. Using the same "hook" position as in Two-Handed Pluck (page 58), pluck at the attacker's thumb area, pulling in a diagonal motion downward across your chest. At the same time, counterattack with a strike to the groin or an elbow to the face.

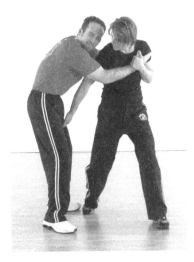

3. Continue with additional counters, turning toward the attacker with elbows and knees.

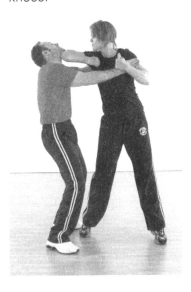

TIPS

Be sure to pluck along your chest, rather than pull away from your body. Pulling away from your body reduces the power of the plucking motion.

CHOKE FROM THE FRONT WITH A PUSH

Self-Defense

A choke with a push represents an added danger. In this case, a regular pluck becomes more difficult because (a) you're being pushed off balance and (b) the shock of a sudden push may cause your hands to fly up and away from your throat.

STARTING POSITION: Passive stance, with an attacker choking you from the front.

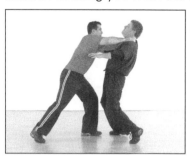

1. To simulate stumbling backwards, lean back, off balance, and then step back on one foot (usually the left foot will be easiest for training purposes). As you step your left foot back, stab your right hand straight up to the sky. Your right bicep/shoulder should be as close to your right ear as possible. This ensures that you defend against the attacker's wrist.

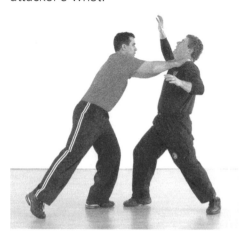

2. Turn sharply to the left. The turn should be about 90°, and should cause pressure against his wrist, not his forearm. This removes the pressure from your throat.

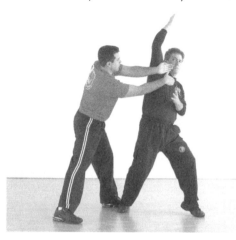

3. Clear the attacker's hands: bend slightly at the knees, delivering a downward vertical elbow strike (#7) with your right hand, while bringing your left hand up in a trapping motion.

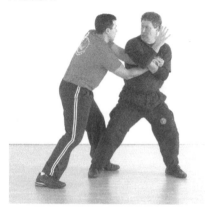

4. Deliver a sideways elbow strike (#2) to your opponent's face. Be sure there is weight behind the attack! Continue with further counters.

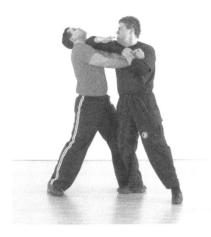

As with any technique, once you've developed skill and comfort performing this from your dominant side, train the opposite side as well.

To simulate reality when being pushed, allow the attack to put you slightly off balance *before* you step back. This feeling of being off balance recreates the surprise of a real attack.

The defense is made by the explosive rotation of the body, *not* by the downward elbow. The elbow simply moves the hands out of the way of your counterattacks.

Self-Defense

The principles of this defense are exactly the same as those for Choke from the Front with a Push (page 64).

STARTING POSITION: Passive stance, with an attacker behind you.

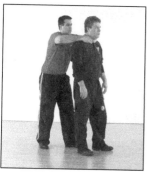

1–2. When the choke and push come from behind, your hands may fly forward (an instinctive motion to prevent a fall). Assuming you step forward with your right foot, bring your left arm up and close to your ear. This ensures that you defend against the attacker's wrist. Turn sharply back toward the attacker. Unlike in the Choke from the Front, this turn should be greater than 90° since, in this case, it brings you around to face the attacker.

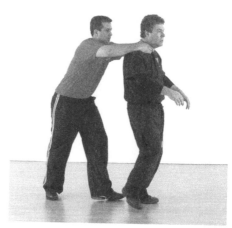

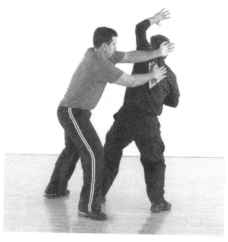

3–5. As you complete the turn, step back with your left (inside) foot—this helps maintain balance against a strong push. Bring your left elbow down to clear the attacker's hands and pin them against your body. At the same time, counterattack with a right punch, followed by multiple left knees.

TIPS

If the push is not strong, stepping back may not be necessary…but in most cases it is.

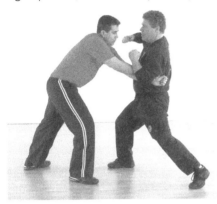

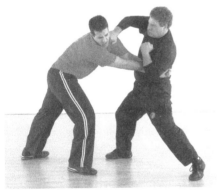

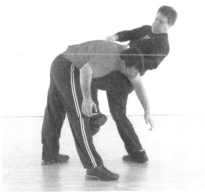

HEADLOCK FROM THE SIDE

Self-Defense

Headlock from the Side represents one of the most common types of holds in schoolyards, street fights, and barroom brawls.

STARTING POSITION: An attacker headlocks you from the side.

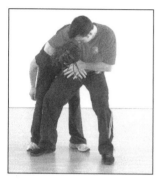

1. As the headlock is made, don't resist the inward/downward pull (assuming you are surprised, you will not be able to resist). Go with it, turning your chin in and down to avoid a choke and limit exposure to a punch. At the same time, strike the attacker's groin with your outside hand (across your bent-over body) while bringing your inside hand up between your head and the attacker's.

2. If the attacker has no hair, go for the eyes and nose, placing your index finger under the nose and your thumb under the chin (avoid fingers over the mouth). Lift the attacker's chin up sharply. Take your inside elbow straight down to your hip while standing up.

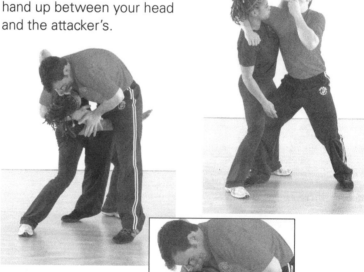

3–4. Deliver counterattacks such as hammerfists or straight punches to the face.

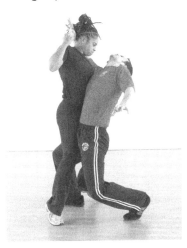

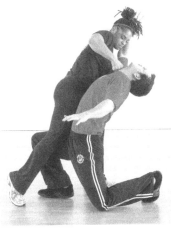

VARIATION: If the attacker has hair, grab the hair (right down to the scalp) at the hairline with your outside hand.

Soft Techniques

This technique should be applied if the other party grabs you on the same/mirror side (e.g., grabs your right hand with his left).

STARTING POSITION: Attacker grabs your right hand with his left hand.

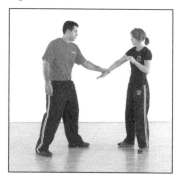

1–2. Move your elbow forward, bending it until it touches (or is very near) your partner's elbow. At the same time, snap your wrist out of the hold, leading with the blade, or thin part of the wrist.

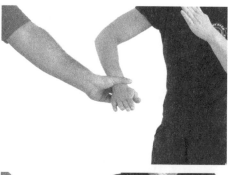

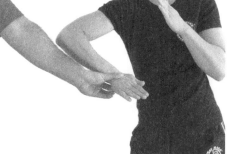

3. Move away, keeping your hands up.

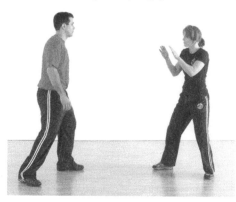

TIPS

It may be necessary to step forward to get close enough to make the release. If a step is necessary, step in with the same-side foot (if your right wrist is held, step with your right foot).

To help remember the technique, think of it as "elbow to elbow."

WRIST RELEASE: OPPOSITE-SIDE HAND (HITCHHIKE OUT)

This technique should be applied if the other party grabs you on the opposite/cross side (e.g., grabs your right hand with his right hand, reaching across your body).

STARTING POSITION: Attacker grabs your left wrist with his left hand.

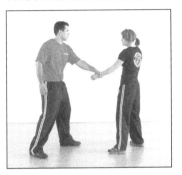

1. Rotate your wrist so that your thumb goes toward the weak part of the grip.

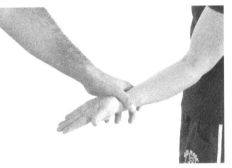

2. Pull in the direction of your shoulder, making a hitchhiking motion.

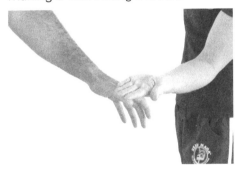

3. Move away, keeping your hands up.

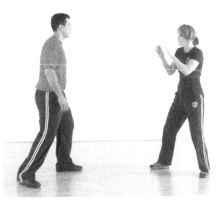

WRIST RELEASE: TWO HANDS HELD HIGH

Soft Techniques

This technique is useful when the other party holds both of your wrists up.

STARTING POSITION: Stand facing your attacker, your elbows bent and hands in front of you.

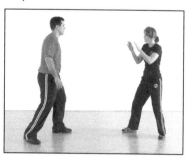

1. As the attacker grabs your wrists, make an inward circular motion with both hands. Move your left hand clockwise and your right hand counterclockwise. As you make the motion, drop your chin to your chest, lowering your face and decreasing exposure to a headbutt, which may be intentional or accidental

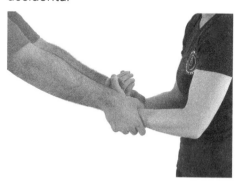

2–3. As your attacker's hands release your wrists, take a small step back to increase the distance. Finish the circular motion so that your hands come outside of his hand and up in a modified fighting stance (in other words, up, but not in any sort of aggressive posture).

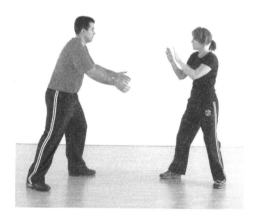

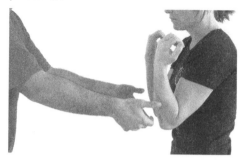

Soft Techniques

Use this technique when the other party holds both your hands down.

STARTING POSITION: Attacker grabs both your wrists from above.

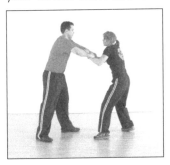

1–2. Bring both hands inward and upward toward your face, making sure to curl your fingers to prevent accidentally poking yourself in the eyes.

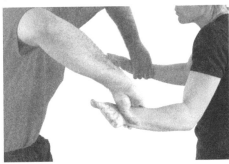

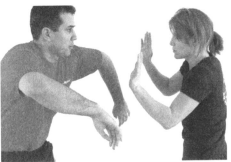

3. Take a small step backward to create more distance.

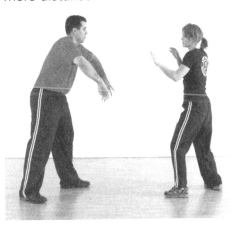

Soft Techniques

STARTING POSITION: Attacker grabs one of your wrists with both of his hands.

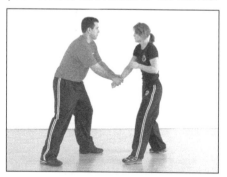

1. With your free hand, reach down and grab your caught hand, making a fist with the caught hand.

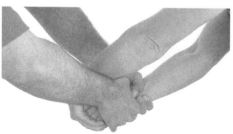

2. Pull the caught fist above the line of your attacker's wrist.

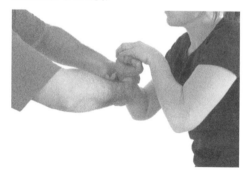

3. Rotate your bent arm sharply, elbow in the air (as in Elbow #1), to release the wrist. Do NOT use the elbow to strike your attacker (remember, this is a soft technique).

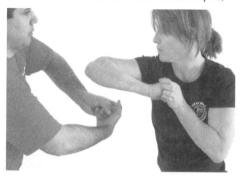

Step away to make distance.

THE POSITION: You're on your back, with head and shoulders up off the ground and chin tucked against your chest. Keep your hands up to protect your face.

Place one foot on the ground near your buttocks. Draw your other knee up close to your chest. Keep your hips off the ground. Once you've taken this position, only a small part of your back and one foot should be touching the ground.

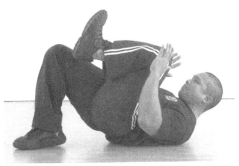

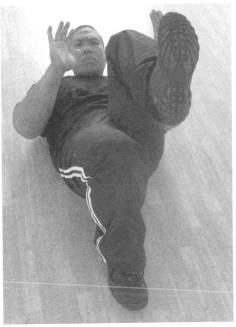

Groundfighting

An attacker may try to scramble around to get at vital parts of your body. Your goal is to keep your feet between your body/head and the attacker. When a correct groundfighting position is taken, only the small of the back and one foot touch the ground, allowing for easier turning.

STARTING POSITION: Back Position.

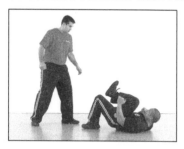

2. Keep the foot closest to the attacker up for kicking purposes—e.g., if the attacker is circling to your left, pull your left foot up and use the right to turn. This makes it more difficult for the attacker to get around your guard.

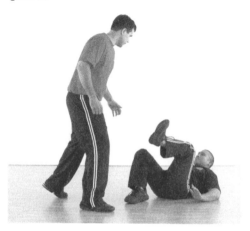

1. Use your planted foot to turn and stop.]

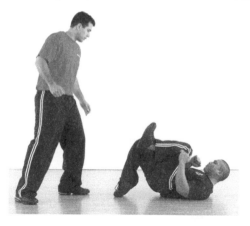

VARIATION: If the attacker is at some distance, you may use your hands for a faster and more controlled turn.

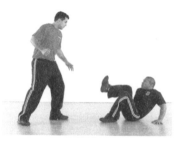

THE POSITION: Lie on one elbow, one hip, and one base leg. Bring your top hand up to protect your face. Hold your top leg up, knee drawn back, ready to kick.

If the attacker is farther off, you may rise onto your lower (base) hand, rather than your elbow, but ONLY if the attacker is farther away.

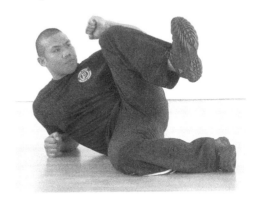

SIDE POSITION: MOVEMENT ON THE GROUND

Groundfighting

An attacker may try to scramble around to get at vital parts of your body. Your goal is to keep your feet between your body/head and the attacker.

STARTING POSITION: Side Position.

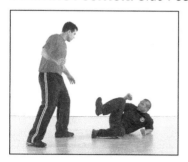

1. If the attacker moves toward your live (front) side, use the base foot to turn and stop.

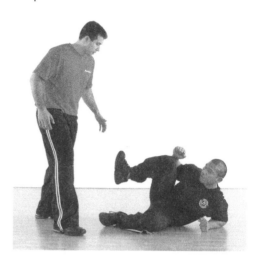

2. If the attacker moves to the dead (back) side, roll to your opposite side and take up the same-side position.

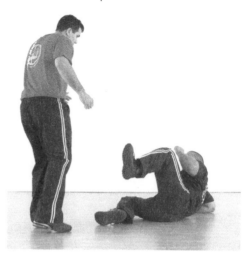

Groundfighting

This kick is more like a stomp (Defensive Front Kick, for those who know it); you make contact with your heel.

STARTING POSITION: Back Position, on the ground.

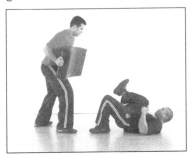

1. Stomp your foot outward horizontally, with power generated by sending your hip out as well—this is most important!

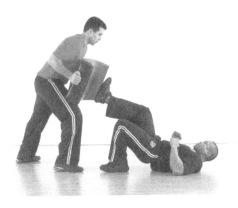

2. At the moment of impact, the only parts of your body touching the ground are your base (planted) foot and your shoulders/elbows.

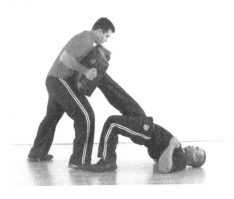

3. Recoil immediately by pulling your knee back to your chest to prepare for another kick.

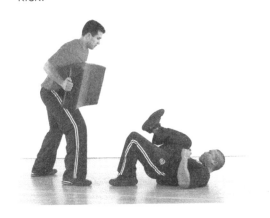

TIPS

When kicking to the shin or knee, turn your foot outward slightly to broaden the kicking surface, giving you the best chance to hit the target.

ROUND KICK FROM THE GROUND

Groundfighting

A round kick while on the ground can be especially useful when an attacker tries to make an "end run" around your guard. As the attacker dodges to the outside of your kicking leg, you roll over and deliver a round kick.

STARTING POSITION: Back Position, on the ground.

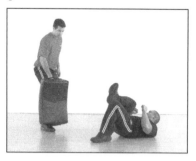

1–2. As you kick, roll your hip over.

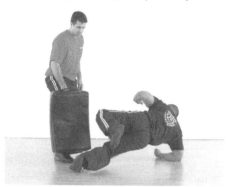

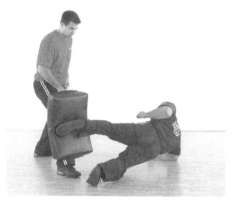

TIPS

For added power, make a slight "scissor" motion with the legs (this simulates the pivoting motion made during a standing round kick).

The kick may be done with either leg, depending on which way the attacker goes. However, the base leg will deliver the strongest round kick (just as the rear leg delivers the strongest standing round kick). As with regular round kick, the kicking surface is the instep or the shin.

A side kick may be necessary after delivering a round kick, or if you end up on your side rather than your back.

STARTING POSITION: Side Position, on the ground.

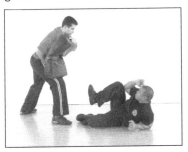

1–2. Send your foot out, extending your hip to generate power, striking with your heel. This is similar to a stomp. Use your base hand (the one closest to the floor) for support and to give a push that helps generate power. You may also use your other hand if the attacker is at a sufficient distance.

Otherwise, that hand should be up in a defensive position. At the point of impact, your heel, knee, hip, and shoulder should all be in line to support the kick.

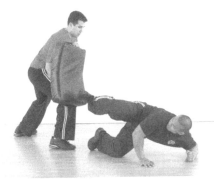

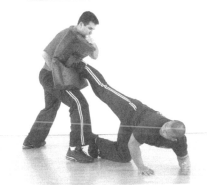

TIPS

This kick may be made to the shins or knees as well as to the midsection.

GETTING UP

Groundfighting

Whenever you're on the ground, your primary goal is to get up. Even good groundfighters must be aware of the dangers of remaining on the ground, since any attacker may have a weapon or an accomplice.

However, getting up is also a tactical decision. If your opponent is standing too close, you will expose yourself to danger while rising. Here we describe the safest way to stand up from a groundfighting position.

STARTING POSITION: On the ground, Back or Side Position (Back Position shown).

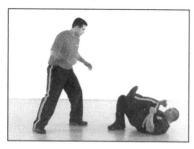

1. Assume your attacker has backed off, perhaps in response to a kick. Bring yourself up to a modified sitting position, keeping your base foot on the ground, your kicking foot up, and one hand on the same side as the base foot up defensively. Your other hand should be on the ground for support. Your kicking foot should be ready to stomp outward, although it will be less powerful in this position. Using your base foot and base hand, lift your hips off the ground.

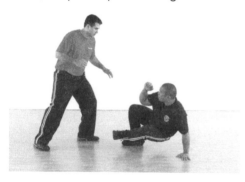

2. Quickly swing your kicking foot back beneath you; be sure to place it behind you, not directly beneath your hips.

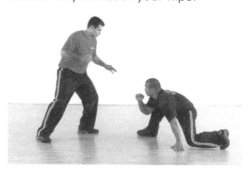

3. Stand up, covering distance backward as you do.

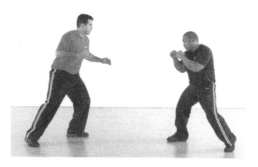

TIPS

When swinging your foot beneath you, move your foot and hip on a diagonal rather than straight back. This is an easier movement. If you cannot lift your hips off the ground using one hand, you can use two. Just be aware that you are less protected this way.

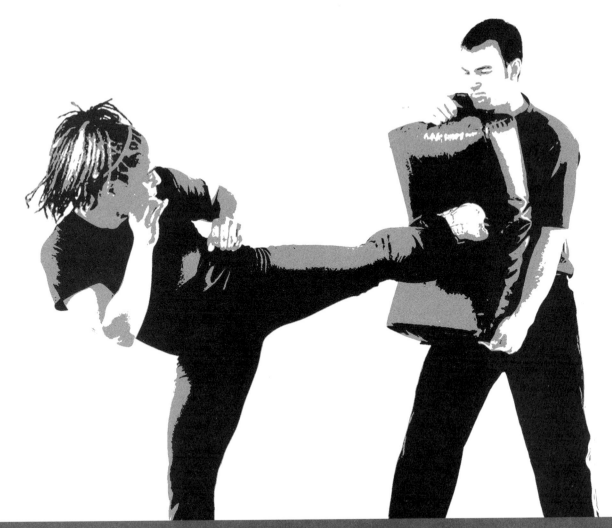

ORANGE
BELT

ORANGE BELT

OVERVIEW

Orange Belt (sometimes termed "Level 2" at a Krav Maga Worldwide school) is the second stage of our curriculum. Here you'll learn basic strikes such as hook punches and uppercut punches, side kicks, and back kicks. You'll also learn how to deal with more common attacks such as bearhugs.

The average training time for this level is six months, assuming you train at least twice a week. At this level, you will see the continuation of the Krav Maga principles. For instance, in Yellow Belt you learned the plucking principle to defend against an attacker's hands on your throat. In Orange Belt, you will apply that same plucking principle to a headlock from behind.

In Yellow Belt, we touched on groundfighting positions, movement, and kicks. In Orange Belt, you will learn how to handle an attacker who is actually on top of you. This is vital because, although we never recommend going to the ground, sometimes in a fight you have no choice and must deal with the situation that is imposed upon you.

The following material is covered at this level:

COMBATIVES

Once you have mastered basic combatives, begin to practice combinations. Any combination that develops your skill in delivering multiple attacks at various angles and heights is beneficial. However, the best combinations are those with practical applications in a fight. Only a few basic combinations are described here. You should feel free to develop your own. As a beginner, it's important to keep focusing as much on the individual techniques as on the combination. Begin with simple combinations and add to them as you become more confident. In all combinations, the strikes should overlap. As you finish one punch, the next should already be traveling toward the target.

DEFENSES AND SELF-DEFENSE

Whenever possible, Krav Maga prefers to defend kicks with the legs. However, in certain instances it may be necessary to make hand defenses instead. This section describes both leg and hand defenses against low kicks. It also touches on several common self-defense scenarios.

CHOKE DEFENSE AGAINST A WALL

These defenses are directly related to Choke with a Push (page 64). However, some points of emphasis are important enough to warrant a separate lesson. Basic knowledge of this type of choke must include the understanding that you may be driven both back into the wall and upward.

HEADLOCK FROM BEHIND

Headlocks from behind represent the most dangerous and immediate threats. All training should consider this danger and the need to respond as quickly as possible. The bar-arm version of the headlock presents a more immediate attack, quickly crushing the windpipe. However, it is moderately easier to defend. The carotid choke takes slightly longer before it is effective, but is more difficult to deal with.

Although we present two headlock defenses, a quick review will reveal that they are essentially the same defense. The only real differences are: a) you have to reach farther back against the carotid choke, and b) the bar arm requires you to pluck down along your chest, whereas the carotid choke requires you to pluck along your shoulder. This plucking angle happens almost automatically.

A Note on Training from a Disadvantage: Although Krav Maga principles always emphasize training from a disadvantage, you should never let anyone get you into a strong headlock (especially the carotid choke) and then try to make the defense. Always respond as early as possible!

BEARHUGS

Bearhugs represent a common type of attack, especially (but not exclusively) against women. You should be aware of the following: Assuming you are surprised, if the attacker's intention is to take you to the ground, you are going to the ground, and you fight from there. None of these techniques (in fact, no technique) will work if you are totally surprised by a "dumping" motion. That's where groundfighting comes in.

These techniques assume that either there is some delay in the dumping technique (caused by you or the attacker's method) or that his intention is to hold you, or take you somewhere, rather than put you on the ground immediately.

Bearhugs are a part of many dangerous scenarios, including being carried into a secluded area or being dumped on the ground. However, while all these situations are problematic, there is no immediate danger presented by the bearhug itself. Unlike chokes, bearhugs themselves do not cause immediate damage. This is important because with no immediate danger to address, Krav Maga's response is to counterattack immediately. If there is even minimal space to operate, Krav Maga simply counterattacks. If the attacker is hugging you close enough to limit even short knees and foot stomps, you must create at least minimal space to operate.

All these techniques will begin with a "space and base" reaction; shift your hips back, body slightly forward, feet in a fighting stance, and center of gravity low.

FALLS

The fight is unpredictable, and you may end up on the ground for a variety of reasons (slipping, being swept, or tripping over obstacles, for example). It is important to learn how to fall safely.

GROUNDFIGHTING

In the Yellow Belt section, we introduced very basic issues on the ground—movement and kicking. In Orange Belt, we include basic grappling skills applied in self-defense situations. These techniques are still basic, and are applied in self-defense situations only. While these techniques do assume very strong attacks, they do not address all the aspects of a ground fight. They are explosive responses to immediate threats, rather than the "chess match" response and counterresponse moves of a larger groundfighting program. As you train in these techniques, be aware that there is a much larger world of groundfighting, and that these techniques are only a small portion related to self-defense.

A Note on Krav Maga's Approach to Groundfighting: Whether you are proficient on the ground or not, our main objective during a groundfight always remains the same: to get up as quickly as possible! During groundfights, you are extremely vulnerable to a second attacker, or to stabs if the opponent produces an edged/pointed weapon.

There are a few basic terms and positions you should know before reading further.

Mount: one person on top, straddling the bottom person.

Guard: the person on the bottom has his legs wrapped around the top person, giving the bottom person some measure of control.

Bobbing and weaving are defensive maneuvers used to avoid punches. They can be extremely handy, even if you're interested only in self-defense.

STARTING POSITION: Left-leg-forward fighting stance.

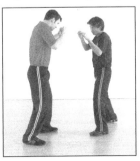

1. Drop straight down by bending slightly at your knees and slightly at your waist, contracting your abs. Keep your hands up!

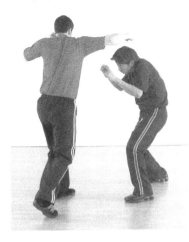

2. Rise up and to the side—NOT straight back up. The movement should be to the dead (i.e., punching) side. In other words, against a left hook, rise up and to your right. Against a right hook, rise up and to your left. Generally, the rising movement should be forward as well as to the side. This puts you in a good position to counterattack.

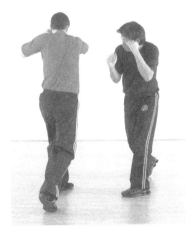

TIPS

Be sure not to look down as you duck. Your eyes should stay up so you can see the fight.

SLIPPING

Combatives

"Slipping" is the act of moving from side to side to avoid a punch (generally a straight or uppercut). Usually you can slip by simply making a small head or body defense.

STARTING POSITION: Left-leg-forward fighting stance.

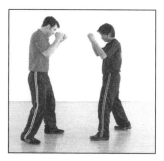

1. As the attacker's punch develops, move your head sideways and in, toward the dead side of the punch (i.e., if a left punch is thrown, move to the right and inward; if a right punch is thrown, move to the left and inward). The motion should be large enough to evade the punch, but still as small as possible (don't exaggerate the motion).

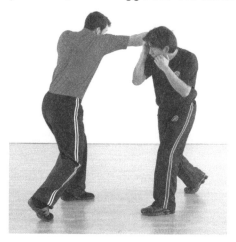

TIPS

Be sure the movement is to the side and INWARD so that you can give counterattacks.

A hook punch is generally suitable when your opponent is close. Rather than punching straight ahead, you bend your elbow and punch around your opponent's defense, aiming at the side of his face or body. Body movement is extremely important when executing a hook punch.

STARTING POSITION: Left-leg-forward fighting stance.

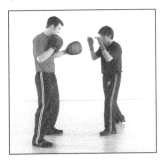

1. Send your left fist forward, bringing your elbow up so that your forearm is parallel to the floor. The elbow should remain bent. As your hand travels to the target, the meaty part (the pinky end of the fist) should remain down. Rotate your left shoulder and hip forward and inward, adding power in the direction of the punch. Make contact with your first two knuckles against the side of your opponent's jaw or body. Pivoting the left (front) foot will add power to a left (or forward) hook punch.

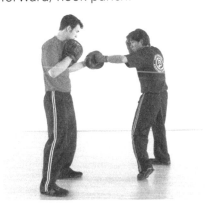

2. Recoil. The fastest way to recover from the hook punch is to simply drop your elbow down. This brings your hand up into a guard position. Then rotate your body back into a normal fighting stance.

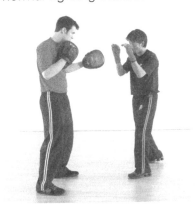

TIPS

For beginners, we emphasize punching with the pinky down to protect the head. Once you have practiced, you can rotate your fist so that the palm faces down.

UPPERCUT PUNCH

Combatives

An uppercut can be thought of as a hook punch at a different angle. Whereas the body rotates inward in the direction of the hook punch, the uppercut punch rotates the body upward.

STARTING POSITION: Left-leg-forward fighting stance.

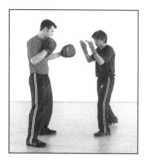

1. Bend slightly at the waist (contracting your abs) and knees. This will drop your center a bit below the target. The amount of bend can be very slight, depending on the height of your opponent. The meaty part of your fist faces outward (toward your opponent's body).

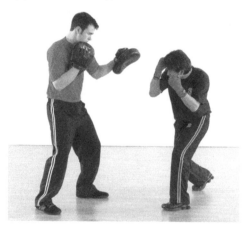

2. Punch out and upward, rotating your left shoulder inward and upward. Keep your elbow close to your body at all times. Do not drop your hand down to your waist—this would expose you to a counterpunch. As your punch rises toward the target, drive your legs upward as well, adding power. Just before contact, rotate your fist so that your palm faces back toward you, which adds torque to the punch.

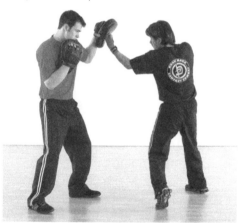

Recoil. The uppercut should punch through the target, then pull back down in a piston-like motion.

TIPS

Use your legs to generate power.

Don't forget you can make a right uppercut as well.

Combatives

This sequence is a rapid combination of left straight punch, right straight punch, and left hook. The attack changes angles, and possibly heights.

STARTING POSITION: Left-leg-forward fighting stance.

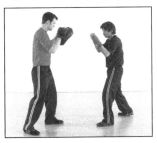

1. Throw a left straight punch. Be sure your left hand comes back to your face as it recoils (don't let it recoil low in preparation for the hook).

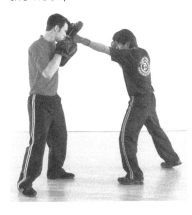

2. As that punch recoils, send a right straight punch, rotating your hips for power but not changing your stance.

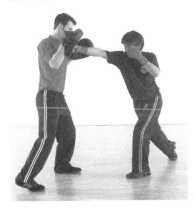

3. As that punch recoils, send a left hook, turning in with your left hip and shoulder.

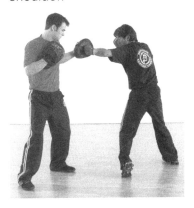

Recoil, returning to fighting stance.

TIPS

The rhythm of the punches should be the same. Avoid a pause between the right punch and the hook. The punches should overlap (i.e., begin the right punch as the left recoils, not after).

Your partner should bring the focus mitt in to about the center of his chest when holding for the hook punch, and tilt the fingers outward slightly, creating a safe angle for your punch.

LEFT/RIGHT/LEFT HOOK/RIGHT UPPERCUT

Combatives

STARTING POSITION: Left-leg-forward fighting stance.

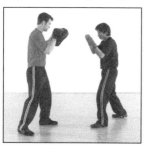

1. Throw a left straight punch. Be sure your left hand comes back to your face as it recoils (don't let it recoil low in preparation for the hook).

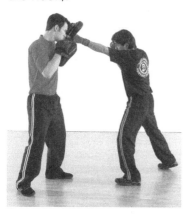

2. As that punch recoils, send a right straight punch, rotating your hips for power but not changing your stance.

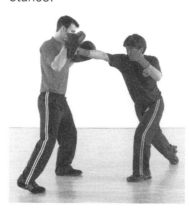

3. As that punch recoils, send a left hook, turning in with your left hip and shoulder. Be sure your right hand recoils to your face after the right straight punch, and NOT low as though preparing for the uppercut.

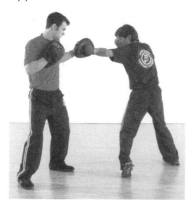

4. Continue with a right uppercut punch.

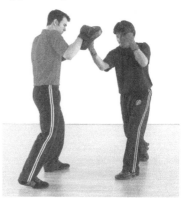

Recoil, returning to fighting stance.

Combatives

This combination simulates throwing a left/right combination, then ducking a left hook and countering with another right punch.

STARTING POSITION: Left-leg-forward fighting stance.

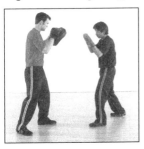

1. Throw a left straight punch. Be sure your left hand comes back to your face as it recoils (don't let it recoil low).

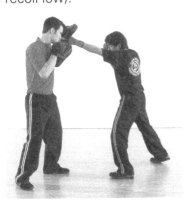

2. As that punch recoils, send a right straight punch, rotating your hips for power but not changing your stance.

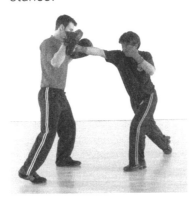

3–4. Keeping your hands up, duck or "bob" to evade a left hook. The ducking motion may move you slightly backward, but this should add more power to the imminent right cross.

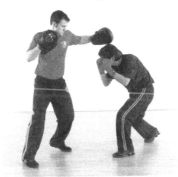

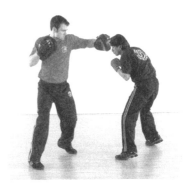

5. Deliver a right cross punch. Make sure there is no delay in delivering it— begin your punch even as you are rising from the bob.

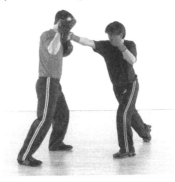

Recoil, returning to fighting stance.

Combatives

STARTING POSITION: Left-leg-forward fighting stance.

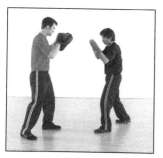

1. Make a strong left jab (don't cheat it in preparation for the elbow). As you throw the jab, make a small advance to set up the elbow. The advance should place you slightly outside your opponent's foot.

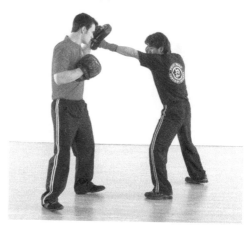

2. Deliver a right elbow strike.

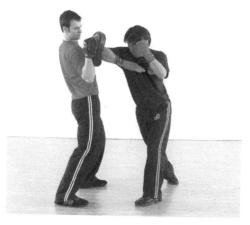

Recover quickly—don't let the elbow strike take you off balance.

This combination is similar to Left/Right/Left Hook/Right Uppercut, except the uppercut is replaced with Elbow #1.

STARTING POSITION: Left-leg-forward fighting stance.

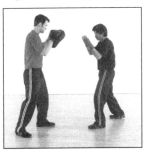

1. Throw a left straight punch. Be sure your left hand comes back to your face as it recoils (don't let it recoil low in preparation for the hook).

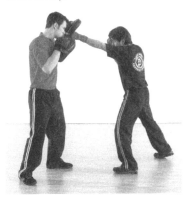

2. As that punch recoils, send a right straight punch, rotating your hips for power but not changing your stance.

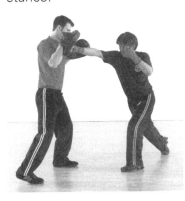

3. As that punch recoils, send a left hook, turning in with your left hip and shoulder. Be sure your right hand recoils to your face after the right straight punch, and NOT low as though preparing for the elbow.

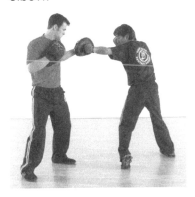

4. Continue with a right elbow strike. Be sure you're close enough to throw the elbow!

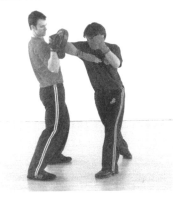

Recoil, returning to fighting stance.

TIPS

The rhythm of the punches should be the same. Avoid any hesitation after the two straights and before the hook/elbow.

Combatives

This combination is unique because it is initiated with an uppercut instead of a straight punch. The right cross can easily be replaced with a right elbow.

STARTING POSITION: Left-leg-forward fighting stance, close in to accommodate the uppercut punch.

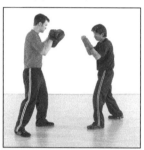

1. Throw a right uppercut.

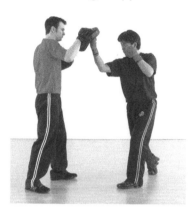

2. Recoil. Make sure your right hand recoils to your face after the punch. Immediately follow with a left hook.

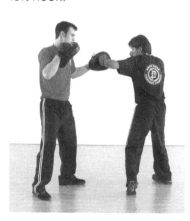

3. Recoil and immediately follow with a right cross.

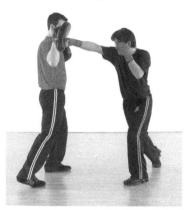

Recoil, returning to fighting stance.

TIPS

The rhythm of the punches should be the same. Avoid any hesitation between them. The uppercut should load the left hook.

Unlike Front Kick to a Vertical Target (page 46), which is designed to penetrate and cause damage, the main purpose of a defensive front kick is to either stop an advancing opponent or to push a close opponent to a greater distance. For this reason, we kick with the whole foot. More surface area means the kick will push more than penetrate.

Caution: *If you are not experienced with kicks, you are in danger of hyperextending your knees. Always practice the kick against a stationary opponent before working against an advancing target. Then begin working against an advancing target that is moving slowly.*

STARTING POSITION: Left-leg-forward fighting stance.

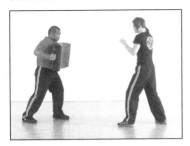

1. Bring your right knee up high, with your toes flexed back (not pointed). Send your foot forward, kicking with the entire sole of your foot (ball to heel). On contact, your knee should still be slightly bent. As with any kick, be sure to extend your hip, which adds reach and power. Also, drive with your base leg for more power.

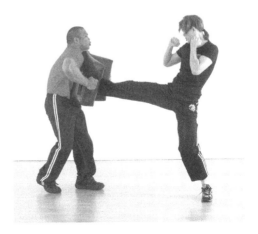

Recoil (either forward or back) quickly.

SIDE KICK

Combatives

Side kick differs from front kick and round kick; it is similar to a stomp. Contact is made with the bottom of the heel.

STARTING POSITION: Passive stance. The target should be directly to your right side.

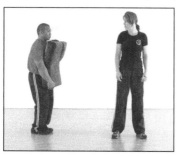

1. Using the right (closest) leg, bring your knee and foot up in front of your body.

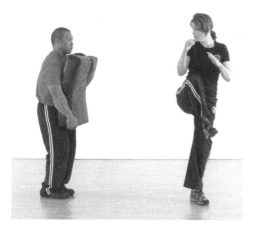

2. Send the bottom of your heel out toward the target while punching your hips in the same direction. For more power and greater height, bend your body over the opposite hip. As your foot moves toward the target, pivot your left (base) foot out so that your left heel points toward the target. Make contact with the bottom of your right heel. Your knee should be slightly bent when you make contact.

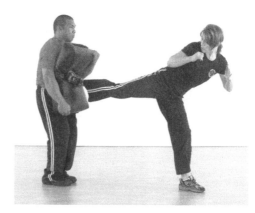

Recoil by making a sharp movement to bring your foot back toward you and down, while straightening your body back to a vertical fighting stance. Turn and face the attacker.

TIPS

Although your shoulders may lean away from the target, your weight should transfer through your hips into the target.

Side kick with advance lets you cover distance and deliver more power.

STARTING POSITION: Passive stance. The target should be directly to your right side.

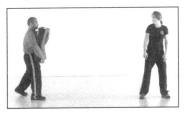

1–2. Burst toward your target with a switch: simultaneously bring your left (back) leg toward the target while bringing your right (close) leg up, knee chambered in front of your body. Your left heel should point at the target.

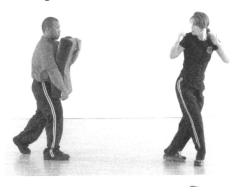

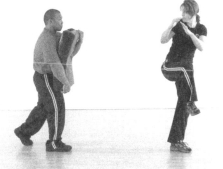

3. Send the bottom of your right heel toward the target while shifting your hips in the same direction. For more power and greater height, bend your body over your left hip. Make contact with the bottom of your heel. Keep a slight bend in your knee when you make contact.

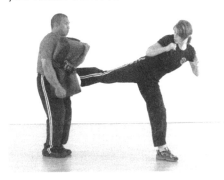

Recoil by making a sharp movement that brings your foot back toward you and down, while straightening your body upright to a fighting stance.

BACK KICK

Combatives

Back kick is more like side kick than front or round kick, in the sense that it's similar to a stomp. You make contact with the bottom of your heel. Practice back kick first while in place, then practice it with a small step.

STARTING POSITION: Passive stance. The target is behind you. First, recognize the threat with a brief, natural glance over your shoulder.

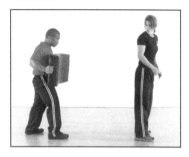

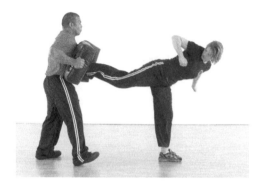

Recoil. As a beginner, you may end up with your back to the target. Once you've mastered the kick, recoil while pivoting on your left (base) foot so that you are facing the target.

1–2. Chamber your right knee in front of you, then send your right foot backward, toes down (not pointed), toward the target. Make contact with your heel going into the target. At the same time, bend your body forward and shift your hips backward into the kick. As you kick, look around your arm, not over your shoulder. If you continue looking over your shoulder, you will be unable to bend and shift your weight into the kick.

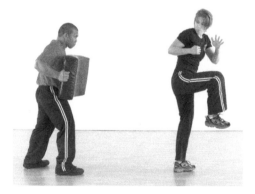

This attack is generally made to an opponent who is behind you. It is useful as one counterattack against Bearhug from Behind (page 192), especially when you're being lifted off the ground.

STARTING POSITION: Passive stance. Your target is behind you.

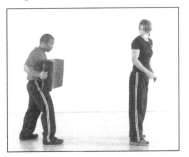

1. Raise your right foot up sharply, with your knee fully bent. Strike with your heel. As much as possible, "pop" your hip up with the help of your left leg for added power.

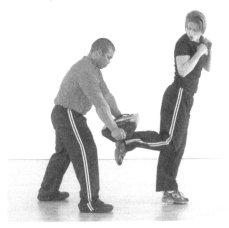

TIPS

Bending your knee sharply allows a full range of motion.

FRONT KICK WITH ADVANCE (FROM A FIGHTING STANCE)

Combatives

You can perform a front kick with an advance when the target is beyond kicking range. As with all advancing kicks, the technique is made using the leg closest to the target. You can start from a neutral stance or fighting stance.

STARTING POSITION: Left-leg-forward fighting stance.

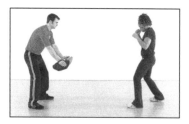

1–2. Bring your right foot forward while simultaneously bringing your left foot up in a front kick. The movement should be made with a "switching" action so that the movements of the front and back leg are almost simultaneous.

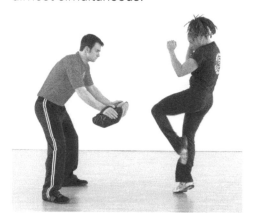

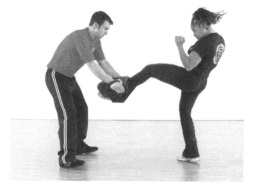

Land with your kicking leg slightly to the outside.

TIPS

Do not step first and then kick. Make the movements as close in time as possible.

Do not jump upward when making the switch; instead, think of traveling forward along the ground.

In this technique, you may kick with either foot.

STARTING POSITION: Neutral stance.

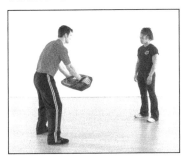

1–2. Burst diagonally forward with one foot while delivering a front kick with the other.

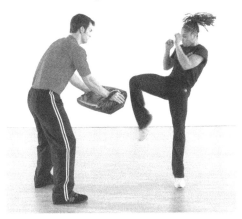

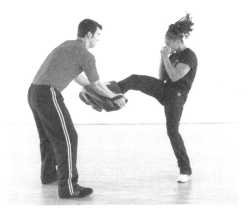

Land with the kicking leg slightly to the outside.

TIPS

DO NOT step first and then kick. The movements should be simultaneous.

SIDE KICK OR BACK KICK/HAMMERFIST

Combatives

After delivering a back kick or side kick (side kick is shown here), the next most immediate weapon is often a horizontal hammerfist with the corresponding hand.

STARTING POSITION: Left-leg-forward fighting stance, with the target to your left side.

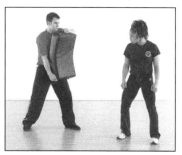

1. Deliver a side kick (or back kick), being sure to recoil your foot after impact.

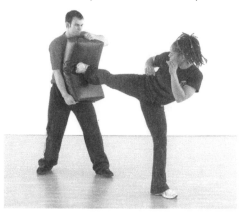

2. As you place your kicking foot down, put it in a position so that you can adequately deliver the hammerfist (in other words, slightly outside and beyond the target).

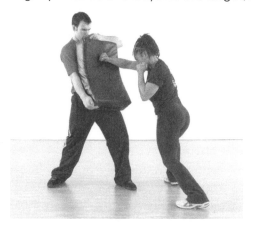

As your foot lands, you should be delivering the hammerfist.

Defenses

Once you have mastered the basic defense against straight punches, add counterattacks that will eliminate or inhibit further attacks.

STARTING POSITION: Left-leg-forward fighting stance.

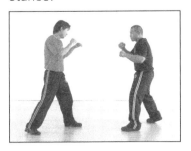

1–2. As your opponent's left punch develops, make an inside defense with your right hand. At the same time, make a left jab to your attacker's face.

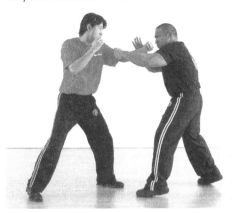

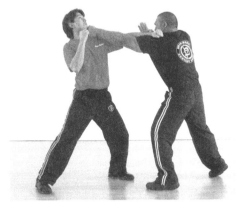

TIPS

Be sure that the body defense accompanying your hand defense takes you forward, allowing you to put strength into your counterattack.

INSIDE PUNCH DEFENSE WITH COUNTERATTACK AGAINST LEFT PUNCH USING LEFT HAND

Defenses

You may have to defend against a left punch with your left hand, either because of an injury to your right hand or by misreading the attack and attempting to recover from a bad position. We never prefer this defense.

STARTING POSITION: Left-leg-forward fighting stance.

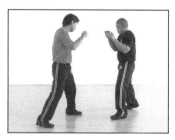

1. As the attacker's left punch develops, with your left hand make a regular inside defense. For additional safety, rotate your wrist sharply as you redirect, trying to stay close to the attacker's wrist. Your defense will now be made against the inside of the attacking hand, rather than the outside as usual. Your hand defense should be accompanied by a body defense. The body defense may be slightly larger than usual to accommodate the possibility that the attacker's elbow may bend around your defense.

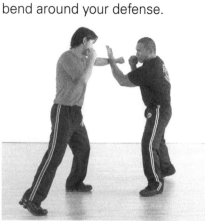

2. Immediately make a hammerfist to the head with your left hand. Be sure to bring your left shoulder up and tuck your chin while making the counterattack. This reduces your exposure to the attacker's right punch.

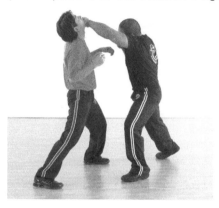

Follow with additional counterattacks.

INSIDE DEFENSE WITH COUNTERATTACK AGAINST RIGHT PUNCH (TWO COUNTERS)

STARTING POSITION: Left-leg-forward fighting stance

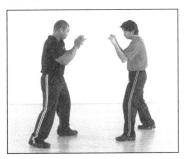

1. As the attacker's right punch develops, make an inside defense with your left hand. At the same time, make a right punch low to the attacker's ribs or stomach. Be sure you recoil the punch.

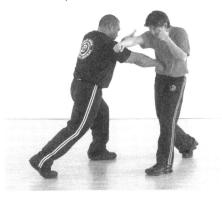

2. Using a "hooking" motion with your left hand, pull the attacker's right hand down slightly.

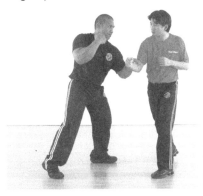

3. Having cleared the right punch, burst in with your feet and make a right punch to the attacker's face.

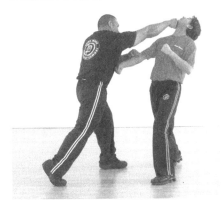

TIPS

If your reaction time is good, you should burst in during the initial defense.

Also, when you hook the attacker's hand, do not pull down too far; only pull down enough to clear his hand out of the way. If you pull too far, your hand will be out of position.

Defenses

Often you will not have time to make a simultaneous defense and counterattack to the body. In this case, a single counterattack must suffice.

STARTING POSITION: Left-leg-forward fighting stance

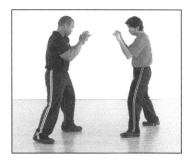

1. As the attacker's right punch develops, make an inside defense with your left hand.

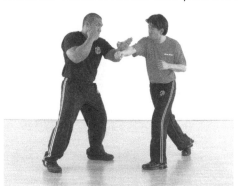

2. Using a "hooking" motion with your left hand, pull the attacker's right hand down.

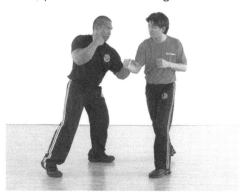

3. Having cleared the right punch, burst in with your feet and make a right punch to the attacker's face. The punch should follow the defense as soon as possible.

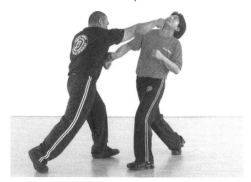

TIPS

When you hook the attacker's hand, do not pull down too far; only pull down enough to clear his hand out of the way. If you pull too far, your hand will be out of position.

Defenses

This defense, which is similar to 360° Defense #3, is made against a hook punch. The attack comes from the outside, and you make your defense with an outward motion to meet it. This defense stops the attack.

STARTING POSITION: Left-leg-forward fighting stance.

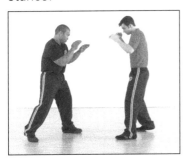

1. As the attacker's punch develops, send your left forearm out to meet it, your hand in a fist. Your elbow should be bent and the back of your hand should face the attack. Make contact as close to the attacker's wrist as possible. Avoid making contact at his elbow—this would allow the punch to come around your defense. As you make the defense, take your head forward and in slightly. This body defense helps avoid a hook punch.

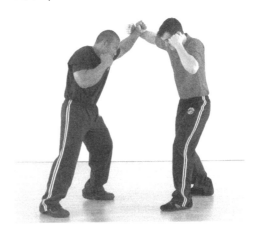

TIPS

Generally, the direction of your defense will be sideways from the shoulder, not forward. You may also simply use 360° Defenses.

DEFENSE AGAINST HOOK PUNCH (COVERING)

Defenses

This technique is a protective covering defense. The advantage is that you leave very little room for an attack to penetrate. If you make the defense well, your forearm and bicep protect your head from injury. The disadvantages are that your ribs are more exposed and you may be a bit slower to counterattack. In addition, the covering defense does not help against a knife attack. For this reason, we generally prefer the extended defense.

STARTING POSITION: Left-leg-forward fighting stance.

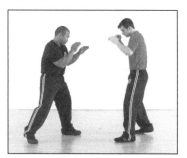

1. As an attacker's left hook punch comes toward you, draw your right fist back so that it's touching the back of your head and your forearm is pressed against the side of your head. Your elbow should point forward, not out at an angle. If it's out at an angle, your chin will be open to uppercuts.

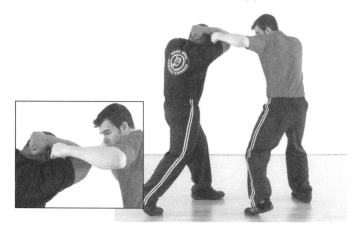

TIPS

Don't just bring your hand back to the side of your head. Your hand itself does not offer protection and can be damaged (remember, we're not wearing boxing gloves on the street). Bring your hand far enough back so that the forearm protects your head.

This defense redirects the uppercut punch. Some of the principles of this defense are the same as for Inside Defenses against Straight Punches: defend with the same-side arm; the movement is inward; the defense redirects the punch.

STARTING POSITION: Left-leg-forward fighting stance.

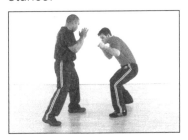

1–2. As an attacker's right uppercut punch begins, move your left (mirror-side) arm inward and upward. Your elbow should lead the motion. Make contact with your arm to the side of the attacker's arm.

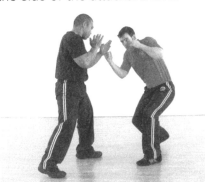

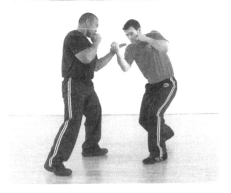

3. Continue the motion inward and upward, rotating your hand and forearm and redirecting the punch away from your face. As you make the arm motion, allow your arm to turn your body and take your head to the outside, creating a body defense.

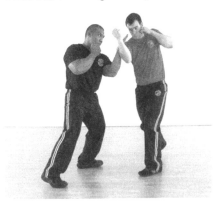

360° DEFENSE WITH COUNTERATTACK

Defenses

"Defend and counterattack at the same time" is a basic principle of Krav Maga. 360° Defenses can easily be made with a simultaneous counterattack.

STARTING POSITION: Left-leg-forward fighting stance.

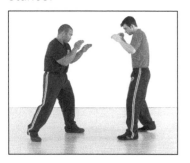

1–2. Defend against any attack with a 360° Defense. Add a punch to the face with your free hand.

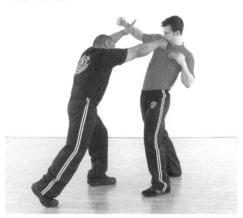

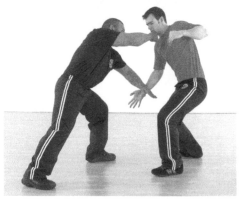

TIPS

The punch should be simultaneous with the defense.

You should train from different states of readiness. If you are early, you should burst forward with your feet. If you are late, you may not have time to move your feet but should still put weight into the defense and counterattack.

This defense is reflexive, and assumes that you are not expecting an attack of any kind and can only respond instinctively. This kick also assumes that your hands are down at your sides at the beginning of the attack.

STARTING POSITION:
Passive/neutral stance.

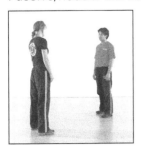

1. As the attacker's kick develops, sweep your left hand across your body. Bend at the waist to reach the kick at an early point. The movement of your arm should be on a diagonal, out and away from your body. Your arm should be stiff and straight, with fingers extended. Make sure your wrist is straight! You do not want to create any angles against the kick.

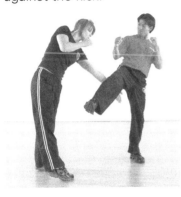

2. With this rigid defending arm, redirect the side of the kicking leg. At the same time, make a body defense, leaning in with your left shoulder, pivoting your right shoulder and hip out of the line of the attack. Your right hand should rise up and across to the left side of your face. This puts your hand in a position to defend either a left or right punch.

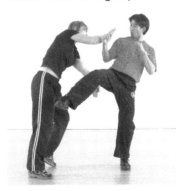

3–4. As you make the defense, burst in. Trap with your right hand, then switch the trap to your left hand to counterattack with your right.

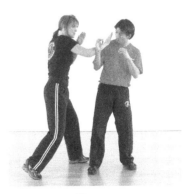

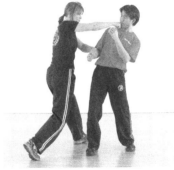

To protect your defending arm from hyperextension, you may bend your elbow slightly.

VARIATION: Alternately, with your right hand, trap the attacker's right hand, counterattacking with the left. This is faster, but may be less comfortable and powerful.

Defenses

This defense is made from a fighting stance when your legs are unavailable to defend, such as when you've lost your balance or your legs are injured.

STARTING POSITION: Left-leg-forward fighting stance.

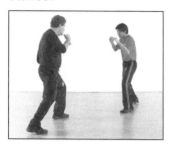

1. As an attacker's kick develops, stab down toward the attacker's knee with your right (back) hand; burst in toward the attacker at a slight diagonal. Keep your elbow in and the meaty part of your hand pointing back toward your body. This ensures that your arm is straight, creating no angle against the kick. Keep your shoulders square to your attacker—turning your right side in will redirect the kick to your body, not away from it. Be sure your left hand is up, protecting your face, in case the kick is followed by an immediate punch. As soon as you've redirected the kick, move your right arm slightly outward, creating a larger defense.

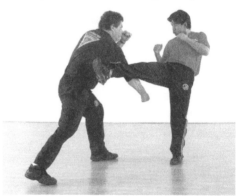

TIPS

If the attacker did not throw a punch, use your left (forward) hand to punch. Make the punch as soon as possible after the kick, and follow with a right punch and additional counterattacks.

If the attacker threw a punch, use your left hand to defend then trap, and counterattack with the right.

This defense can be made to the live or dead side, using either hand. However, it is generally easier to defend on your live side because it makes the body defense simpler (the hips are already turned). However, these two options are not always offered at the same time.

STARTING POSITION: Left-leg-forward fighting stance.

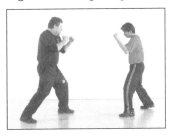

1. As the attacker's kick develops, reach out with your right hand toward the rising kick; try to avoid offering an angle to the kick that could cause you to be kicked on the forearm.

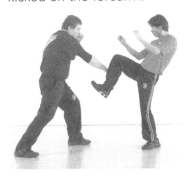

2–3. As your hand passes the kick, pluck backward, letting your elbow and forearm slide tight along your body. As you pluck or pull at the foot, let that motion pull your body forward (with your left side leading), making a body defense; burst in with your feet. If you pluck to your live side, you will burst forward in a regular fighting position.

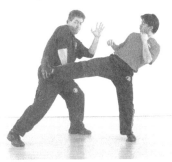

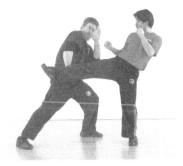

4. Counterattack with your right hand.

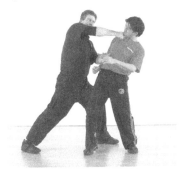

TIPS

This technique must be performed quickly; your defending hand moves in a quick "pickpocket" motion.

Defenses

This is a redirecting defense.

STARTING POSITION: Left-leg-forward fighting stance.

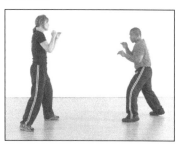

1. As the attacker's kick develops, bring your left (forward) forearm across your face and upper body, parallel to the floor. Your hand may be in a fist—rotate it so that the meaty part of your hand makes the deflection. As you make the hand defense, add a small body defense by moving your left shoulder in and turning your right shoulder slightly out. Be sure your weight stays in the fight!

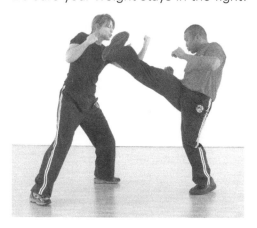

2. Continue with counters: either a hammerfist with the left hand (after making the defense) or a right cross (or both).

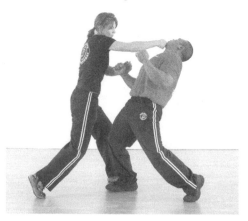

STARTING POSITION: Left-leg-forward fighting stance.

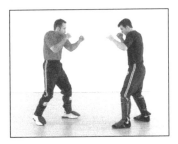

1. As the attacker makes a right round kick, bring your left knee up, angled out at about 45° (your knee should point toward the incoming kick). Your toes should be pulled up (this helps to flex the muscles along the calf, offering at least some protection for the shin). In case the kick comes high instead of low, have your left arm up in a defensive position with the elbow touching your left (defending) thigh, making a complete wall from foot to fist.

2. Try to make the defense with the middle or upper portion of your shin against the attacker's ankle. As the kick makes contact, let your shin "give" slightly, creating a shock absorber effect. Then pop your foot back out, pushing the kicking foot away.

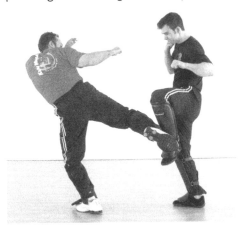

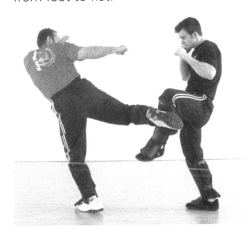

TIPS

If the attacker delivers a left round kick low, you may of course use the other (rear) leg. However, some left round kicks target your forward leg, so you may use your forward leg to defend. The rule of thumb: Use the closest leg to defend!

Defenses

STARTING POSITION: Left-leg-forward fighting stance.

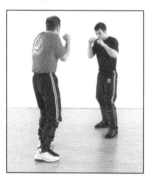

1. As the attacker's kick develops, pivot on the ball of your left foot so your knee points toward the incoming kick. Flex your quadriceps (thigh muscles) and bend your knee slightly. Take the impact on the strong thigh muscle. Do not take the kick on the side of your leg, which is more painful.

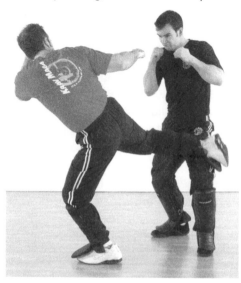

STARTING POSITION: Left-leg-forward fighting stance.

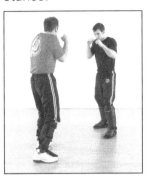

1. As the attacker's kick develops, lift your left knee almost as though preparing to give a side kick (but don't chamber quite that high).

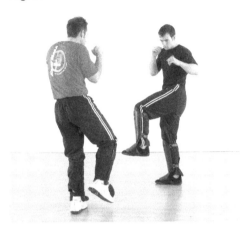

2. With your toes turned inward, stomp on the attacker's shin or, if you meet the attack very early, his knee.

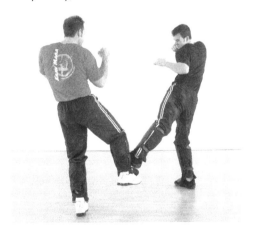

TIPS

This defense is very effective, but it assumes you see the kick early or in time.

Defenses

STARTING POSITION: Left-leg-forward fighting stance.

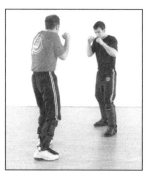

1. As the attacker's kick develops, bring your left knee up and across your groin. Your knee should not be too bent (in other words, the foot should be almost right beneath the knee). If it is bent, this creates an angle against the front kick, which you don't want. Your shin should brush the side of the attacking foot or leg. As you make contact, redirect the kick away from your groin, allowing the motion to continue, if possible.

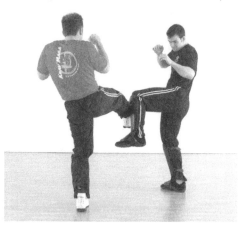

Practice the defense against Choke from the Front with a Push (page 64).

STARTING POSITION: Passive stance, back to a wall, with an attacker choking you from the front, pinning you to the wall.

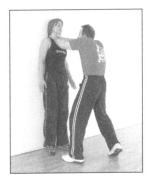

1. Stab your left hand straight up to the sky. Your left bicep/shoulder should be as close to your left ear as possible.]

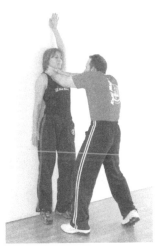

2. Turn sharply to the right, dropping your right shoulder down so that your body and neck stay against the wall.

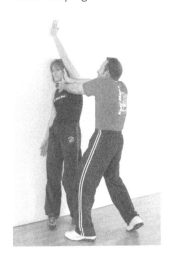

3. Clear the attacker's hands: bend slightly at the knees, delivering a downward vertical elbow strike (#7) with your left arm, while bringing your right hand up in a trapping motion.

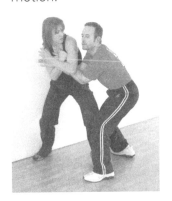

4. Deliver an upward angled elbow strike (#2) to your opponent's face. Be sure there is weight behind the attack! Continue with further counters.

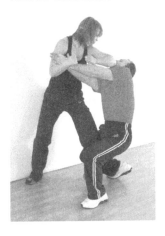

TIPS

Dropping your shoulder is vital. If you keep your shoulder up as you turn, you will increase the pressure on your throat, which is not good. Drop your shoulder as you rotate and the hands will come off your throat smoothly.

Self-Defense

All the principles of Choke from Behind with a Push (page 66) apply.

STARTING POSITION: Passive stance, facing a wall, with an attacker choking you from behind.

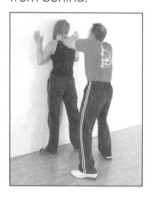

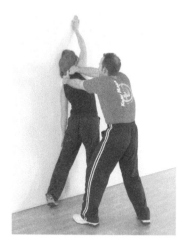

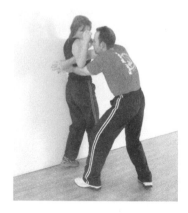

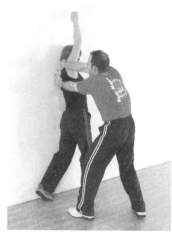

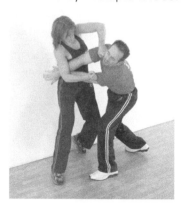

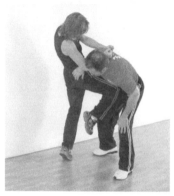

1–2. Raise one hand up along the wall and turn sharply back toward the attacker. Unlike in Choke from the Front (page 121), you do not have the option of defending to either side. Your face will be turned to one side or the other, and you must pivot in that direction. As you turn, drop the shoulder on the non-defending side down so that your body and neck stay against the wall.

3. Bring your elbow down to clear the attacker's hands and pin them against your body.

4–5. At the same time, counterattack with a punch, followed by multiple knees.

As the attacker chokes and begins to pull, in training let yourself be pulled off balance before reacting (to simulate a real situation).

STARTING POSITION: Passive stance, with an attacker choking and pulling from behind.

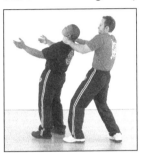

1–2. Immediately make the plucking motion (this is instinctive) as though performing a regular Choke from Behind defense. At the same time, you may take a small step backward with one foot. This is also instinctive, to keep your balance. In training, be sure the step is small, as a large step will be unlikely when you are surprised.

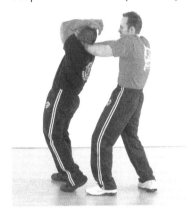

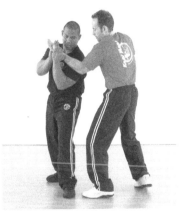

steps 3–5 continued on next page

Self-Defense

continued from previous page

3. As you pluck, step then pivot sharply toward your back foot, keeping hold of the attacker's hand on that side.

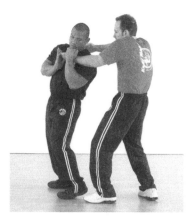

4. As you pivot, burst forward with the other foot and release the attacker's opposite hand. Bring your hand over and press against the pinky side of the attacker's hand with the heel of your palm (see close-up). Keep his hand relatively square in front of your body.

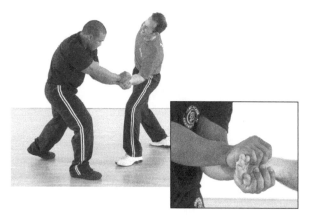

5. As you complete the large step, make a front kick or, if appropriate, a round kick (using the ball of the foot if possible) to the attacker's groin. This can be followed by a Side Kick to the knee, or additional attacks.

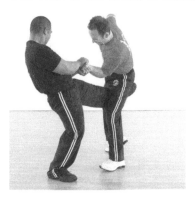

TIPS

The bursting motion you perform while pivoting (Step 4) serves three purposes: 1) it increases pressure on the attacker's wrist; 2) it helps you regain your balance; and 3) it gets you farther away from the attacker's other weapons.

Here, the attacker lays his forearm across your throat to crush it.

STARTING POSITION: Passive stance, with an attacker applying a headlock from behind.

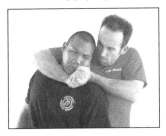

1. If possible, turn your chin away from the elbow and toward the attacker's joined hands. Drop your chin down. Send both hands up and backward to the attacker's joined hands. Note that both your hands go over one shoulder; your closer hand can lead the other slightly. Send your hands back far enough to ensure they'll reach the attacker's hands (this has the potential benefit of scratching the attacker's eyes).

2. Using the plucking motion, pull your hands sharply down along your chest (note that the motion is explosive); turn your inside shoulder sharply inward to create additional space.

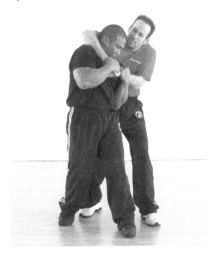

steps 3–5 continued on next page

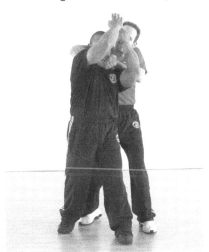

HEADLOCK FROM BEHIND (BAR ARM)

Self-Defense

continued from previous page

3–4. Slide your head out of the opening.

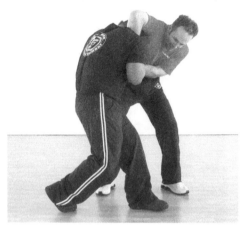

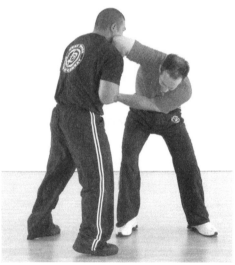

5. Make immediate counterattacks with kicks, knees, fists, or whatever is convenient.

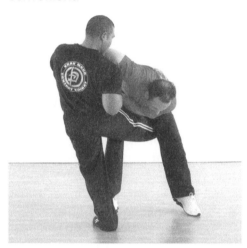

TIPS

By plucking down along your chest, you will be plucking 90° against the choke. This knowledge becomes important for an overall understanding of the defense, but need not be studied initially.

Both hands may travel at the same time, but the hand closest to the attacker's hands may arrive first. If so, the second hand should arrive immediately to help.

Self-Defense

Although the carotid choke presents a greater danger than the bar arm, the defense is essentially the same. The attacker reaches around your neck, putting your throat in the crook of his elbow. In this position, he can put pressure on the carotid arteries at the sides of your neck, stopping blood flow to your brain and putting you to "sleep."

Be aware that an experienced attacker, given time, can create problematic attacks by crossing his rear arm against the back of your neck, increasing pressure and hiding the weak part of the choke. For this reason, awareness and immediate reaction become the best defenses.

STARTING POSITION: Passive stance, with an attacker applying a choking headlock from behind.

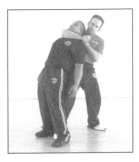

1. Immediately turn your chin away from the elbow and toward the attacker's joined hands. Drop your chin down.

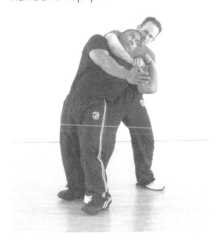

2. Send both hands up and backward to the attacker's joined hands. Note that both your hands go over one shoulder. Send your hands back far enough to ensure they'll reach the attacker's hands (this has the potential benefit of scratching the attacker's eyes).

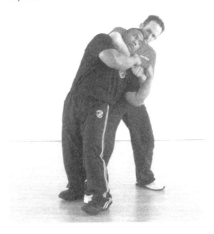

steps 3–6 continued on next page

Self-Defense

continued from previous page

3. Using the plucking motion, pluck along your own shoulder, which makes the pluck 90° to the hold (note that the motion is explosive); turn your inside shoulder sharply inward to create additional space.

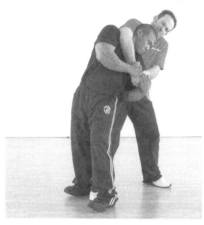

4–5. Slide your head out of the opening.

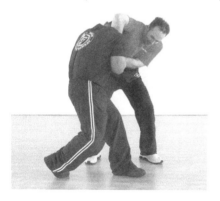

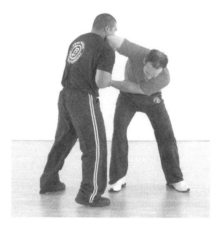

6. Make immediate counterattacks with knees, fists, or whatever is convenient.

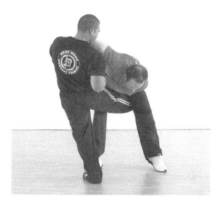

TIPS

As you reach, your near hand may arrive first (in fact, against the carotid choke, it probably will). This is fine, and will often ensure that you reach far enough back. Just be sure your second hand arrives in time to help.

With your arms free, if there is space to operate, you have weapons available but you are in serious danger of a takedown. The attacker has "underhooks," which many wrestlers use to initiate takedowns. You must prevent this type of attack while allowing maximum power in counterattacks.

STARTING POSITION: Passive stance while an attacker bearhugs you from the front, leaving your arms free.

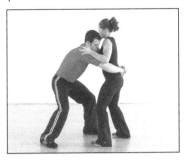

1. As the attacker applies the bearhug, kick your hips and feet back and lower your center of gravity, making yourself harder to lift (space and base). Reach around his arms to put both of your hands on (or near) his hips.

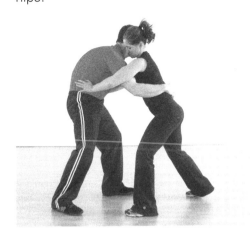

2. Deliver knee strikes immediately.

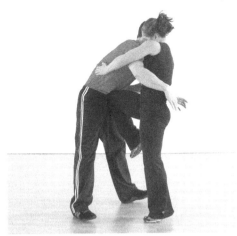

When appropriate, release your hands and continue to counter or disengage and make distance.

TIPS

For additional defensive tactics, see Bearhug from the Front with Arms Free—Leverage on the Neck (page 130).

If the attacker is large, it may be difficult to get your hands near his hips. We rely on the knee to keep him away. We also rely on the next technique.

BEARHUG FROM THE FRONT WITH ARMS FREE (LEVERAGE ON THE NECK)

Self-Defense

This variation is possible as a follow-up to the previous defense, or when space restrictions or imbalance prevent you from delivering knees.

STARTING POSITION: Passive stance while an attacker bearhugs you from the front, leaving your arms free.

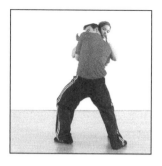

1. As the attacker squeezes you in, his head will generally turn to one side or the other against your chest. With your opposite-side arm, reach around the attacker's head, grabbing the hair at the temple. If the attacker has no hair, reach slightly farther and grab along the nose ridge while pressing into the eyes.

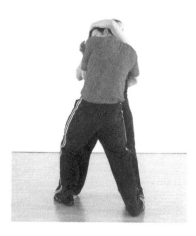

2. Twist the attacker's face away. His chin should rotate away from your body. You may use your other hand to aid this motion by placing the heel of your palm against his chin and pushing.

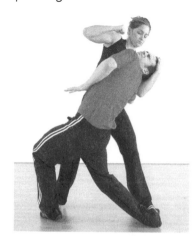

3. As the attacker is peeled away, step out with your foot, allowing him to drop down. Counterattack with straight punches or hammerfist punches.

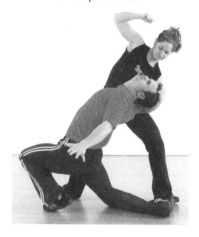

TIPS

It is also possible to use the same-side hand and drive the webbing between your thumb and finger under his nose to drive the attacker's chin up.

BEARHUG FROM THE FRONT WITH ARMS CAUGHT (WITH SPACE)

If there is space (i.e., if your feet are stable and there is a small gap between you and the attacker), counterattack.

STARTING POSITION: Passive stance while an attacker bearhugs you from the front, trapping your arms but leaving some space.

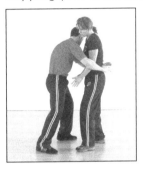

1. Jam the heels of your palms against the attacker's hips to prevent his hips from getting closer to you.

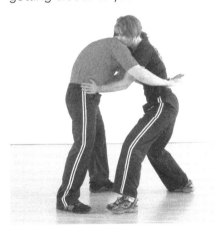

2. Deliver knees to the groin or midsection.

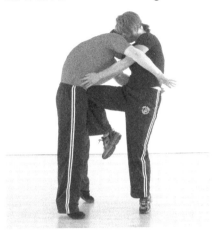

3. Immediately, when any space is created, bring your inside hand up and lay your forearm across the attacker's neck to control his body (preventing him from shooting in).

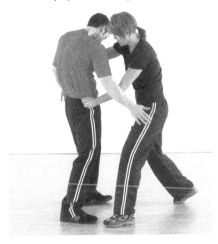

TIPS

If there is space, other counterattacks can include foot stomps or kicks to the groin.

Self-Defense

In order to counterattack, you must create space.

STARTING POSITION: Passive stance while an attacker bearhugs you from the front, trapping your arms.

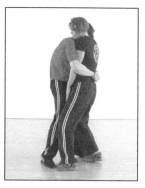

1. As the bearhug is made, send one or both hands to the attacker's groin. This should cause the attacker to shift his hips backward, creating space.

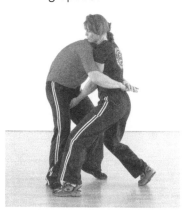

2. Jam the heels of your palms against the attacker's hips to prevent his hips from getting closer to you.

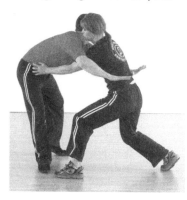

3. Deliver knees to the groin or midsection.

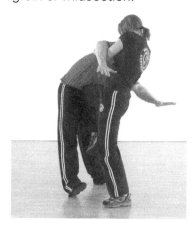

4. Immediately, when any space is created, bring your inside hand up and lay your forearm across the attacker's neck to control his body (preventing him from shooting in).

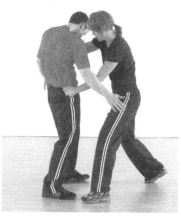

To allow your hand to strike his groin, shift your hips slightly to one side and strike with the open-side hand. We say "strike" but of course you can also grab, twist, and tear. This may get the reaction you want!

STARTING POSITION: Passive stance while an attacker bearhugs you from behind, leaving your arms free.

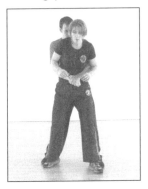

1. When grabbed from behind, immediately drop your weight down and forward to make yourself more difficult to lift (space and base).

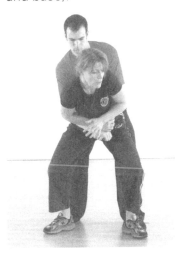

2–3. Send elbow strikes backward to the attacker's face. Always send a "one-two" combination using both elbows.

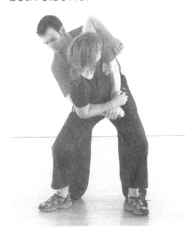

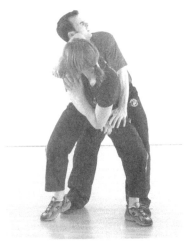

4. If your elbows create space, turn and continue with strikes.

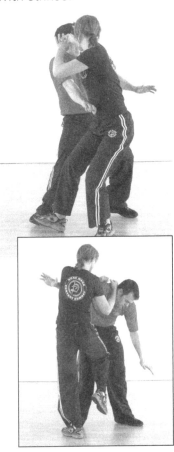

If your elbow strikes don't create space, continue with additional strikes, including stomps to the feet, heel strikes to the shins, and uppercut back kicks to the groin.

Self-Defense

STARTING POSITION: Passive stance while an attacker bearhugs you from behind, trapping your arms but leaving some space.

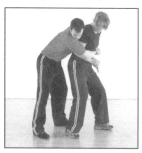

1. When the attacker grabs, immediately drop your weight to make yourself more difficult to lift.

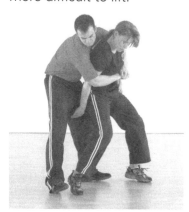

2. Use your arms to create space by striking at the groin—the attacks should cause damage but also create movement so you are hard to hold.

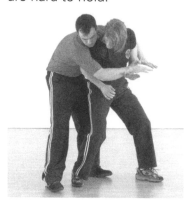

3–4. Make additional counterattacks such as stomps, heel kicks to the attacker's shin, elbows to the body, and uppercut back kicks to the groin. Be sure to make yourself extremely difficult to hold onto by shifting and struggling against the hold.

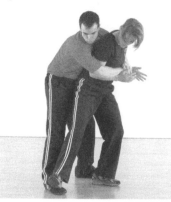

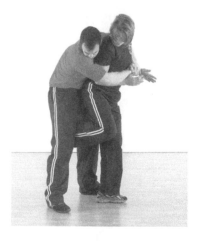

5. As soon as enough space is created, pivot to face the attacker and continue counterattacking.

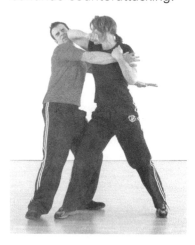

BEARHUG FROM BEHIND WITH ARMS CAUGHT (NO SPACE)

The principles of this technique are exactly the same as those in Bearhug from the Front with Arms Caught—with Space (page 131).

STARTING POSITION: Passive stance while an attacker bearhugs you from behind, trapping your arms.

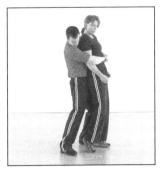

1. When the attacker grabs, immediately drop your weight to make yourself more difficult to lift. Note that this may be more difficult, assuming you've already been squeezed in fairly tight.

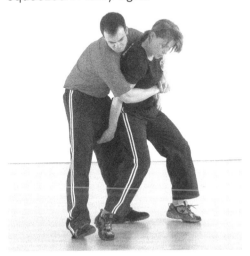

2. Shift your hips and send one hand backward to strike the assailant's groin, causing a backward shift in his hips to create space.

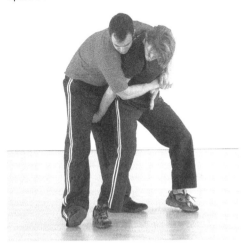

3. Once space is created, continue as in Bearhug from Behind with Arms Caught-with Space (page 134).

BACK FALL BREAK

Falls

As you fall, your goal is to absorb the impact along your palms and forearms, and along the broad muscles in your upper back, while protecting your head and lower back from injury.

STARTING POSITION:
Standing.

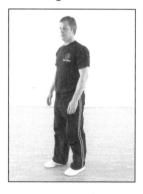

1. When first learning fall breaks, you may want to start by squatting low.

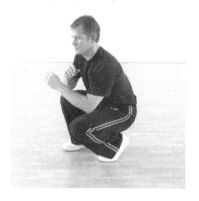

2. Fall backward, leading as much as possible with your upper body and pulling your hips up. Tuck your chin and keep your teeth together. This protects your head and neck, and avoids the risk of biting your tongue.

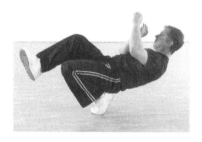

3. As you reach the ground, strike it hard with your palms at about a 45° angle. Do not lead with your elbows. If they strike the ground, you may seriously damage them.

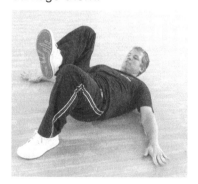

4. Immediately recoil your hands into a fighting position.

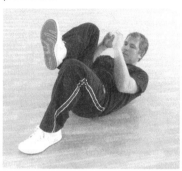

Side fall break follows all the same principles as back fall break. The assumption is that, due to the nature of the takedown or your body position, your fall is to one side of your body and you are limited to the use of one hand. As you fall, your goal is to absorb the impact along one palm and forearm, and along the broad muscles in your upper back, while protecting your head and lower back from injury.

STARTING POSITION:
Standing.

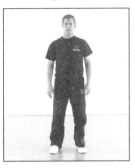

1. As a training method, to fall to your right, shoot your right leg straight out and fall with your right side leading toward the floor. Lead as much as possible with your upper body and pull your hips up. Tuck your chin and keep your teeth together. This protects your head and neck.

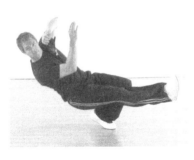

2. As you reach the ground, strike it hard with your palm at about a 45° angle. Do not lead with your elbow. If it strikes the ground, you may seriously damage

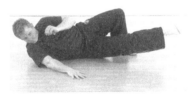

3. Immediately recoil into a fighting position. Because of the nature of the fall, you may end up in a "sideways" groundfighting position (page 77).

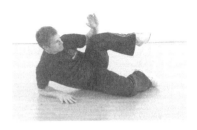

TIPS

Often when being taken down in a wrist lock ("cavalier") or some sort of joint lock, the body will twist or spin toward the floor. As you make the fall break, allow the leg on the falling side to bend. This helps absorb more impact just after the strike.

Groundfighting

Being on your back with someone straddling you (mounted) and throwing punches at you is the second worst position you can be in (the worst is the same position, except you're face down). However, it is a fairly common position to be in when mistakes are made earlier in the fight. While there is no magical solution to this problem, there are tactics that can inhibit or at least reduce the number of punches thrown. This technique introduces the idea of bucking your hips, which is a fundamental principle in ground defense.

STARTING POSITION: On the ground, face up, with an attacker straddling you.

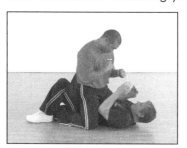

1. If you are mounted, you still need to establish a good position. Keep your elbows down and your hands near your face. Jam your elbows into your opponent's thighs or knees to prevent him from sliding up. Good grapplers will try to get their knees up under your arm pits. This inhibits your arm movement and gets the attacker away from your hips. You want the opposite: You want your elbows down and the attacker on your hips, where you can buck him off.

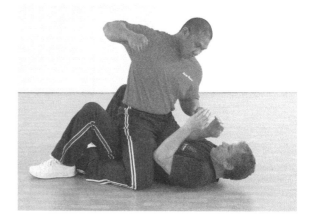

2–3. As punches start flying, buck your hips to throw the attacker off balance. Your hip should move upward and toward your head. Imagine that there is a tennis ball on your stomach and you want to pop it to someone standing at your head. The attacker will probably have to "base" himself out with his hands. This gives you a chance to trap and roll (see next exercise), and at the very least it stops him from punching. Be sure your hands stay up—not every moment of bucking will inhibit a punch, and you should still try to defend against the punches with inside and outside defenses.

Some attackers will lean their weight backwards like rodeo cowboys to maintain balance. While this inhibits your ability to trap and roll, it does reduce their punching ability since they can't punch with much power when their weight is back.

When attempting this technique or the variation, do not reach out with your arms or straighten them, which would expose you to an arm bar.

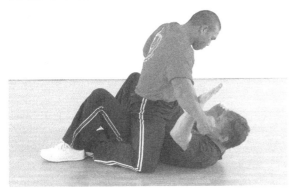

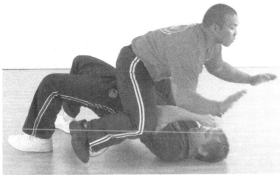

VARIATION: It is also possible, if the attacker is fairly close to you, to try to "hug" him tightly to your chest. This inhibits his punching ability. From there, work toward a trap and roll (page 140).

TRAP AND ROLL AGAINST FULL MOUNT

Groundfighting

Although introduced here in a specific context, the principles of "trap and roll" can be applied to a variety of situations. The basic concept is that a mounted attacker must "base out" with both arms and legs. If you trap the arm and leg on one side, the person can be rolled.

STARTING POSITION: On the ground, face up, with an attacker straddling you.

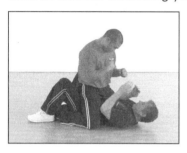

1. Buck your hips to make the attacker base out.

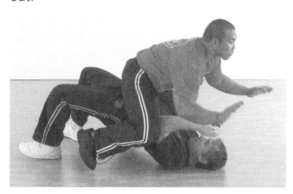

2–3. With one arm, reach out to trap one of his arms. You can reach either over (trapping from the inside out) or under (trapping from the outside in). Generally, reaching over the arm makes for a better hold but may take longer to execute. Be sure that you trap the arm above the elbow. Using your leg, trap the attacker's leg on the same side as the arm—as much as possible at the same time as your arm trap.

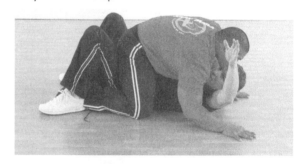

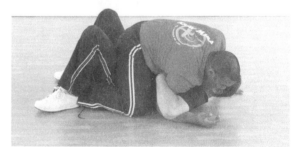

4–7. Buck your hips upward toward your head. At the end of this motion, roll your hips over toward *the trapped side. Drive over with your feet to end up on top, striking as you go. Your goal should be to deliver an elbow to the face, but if the attacker's resistance makes that impossible, deliver groin strikes. (See later techniques for escaping from this position.)*

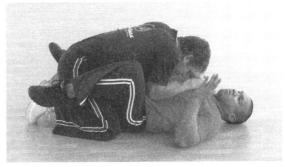

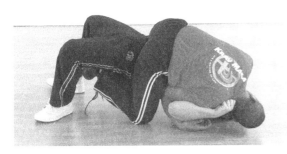

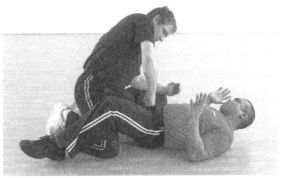

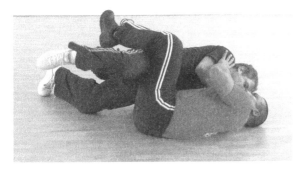

(See later techniques for escaping from this position.)

TIPS

Proficient groundfighters will make it difficult to trap an arm. If you cannot get the arm in a single try, continue bucking your hips, forcing them to base out. Remember that, at the very least, as long as they are basing out, they are not punching you. Also, any method you can create to trap the arm is fine: grab his clothing, grab his wrist with two hands.

SAFETY COMMENT!

When practicing with a partner, be sure the attacker turns his palm up as soon as his arm is caught. This prevents wrist injuries when he is rolled over.

CHOKE WITH ATTACKER IN MOUNT

Groundfighting

STARTING POSITION: On the ground, face up, with an attacker straddling and choking you.

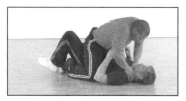

1–2. Address the danger immediately by making the same plucking motion as Choke from the Front (page 58). Be aware that because of interference from the ground, you won't have the same range of motion. Just as with the choke defense from a standing position, pin the hands to your shoulders as you finish the pluck. At the same time, bring one foot up to trap the attacker's leg.

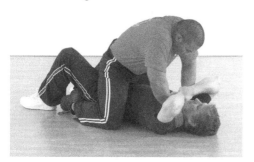

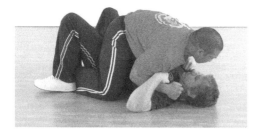

3. Pluck, and punch your hips up to throw the attacker up and toward one shoulder (the shoulder on the same side as the leg trap). Because you have trapped his hands, this should inhibit his ability to "base out."

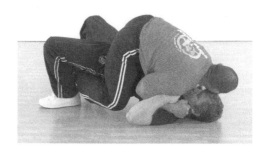

4–8. Roll the attacker over and immediately counterattack. Your goal should be to deliver an elbow to the face. If your movement is inhibited by the attacker's resistance or your technique, groin strikes are possible.

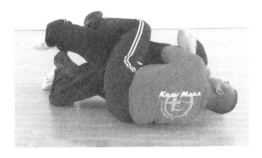

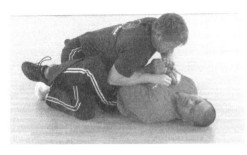

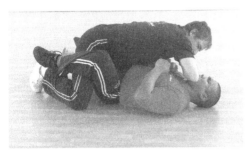

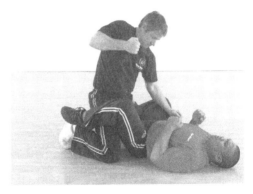

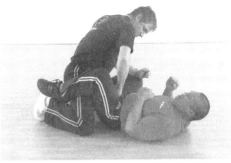

Get up as soon as possible (see later techniques for escaping from this position).

TIPS

The plucking and hip thrust are not made in interrupted stages. The movements are explosive and come almost simultaneously.

Note that a more experienced grappler may apply a more dangerous version of this attack designed not to choke you in a headlock, but to put pressure on your neck, or to crush your face with his chest.

HEADLOCK WHILE MOUNTED

Groundfighting

Another fairly common attack, especially among less-experienced grapplers, is a headlock from the mounted position. In rape or sexual assault scenarios, versions of this attack are made when the attacker wants to taunt the defender, whisper to him/her, or kiss. This technique also works when the attacker is actually choking with his hands, but his elbows are very bent to allow him to get close. The defense against this attack is a simple trap-and-roll.

STARTING POSITION: On the ground, face up, with an attacker straddling you and holding you in a headlock.

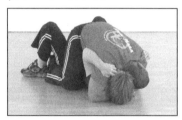

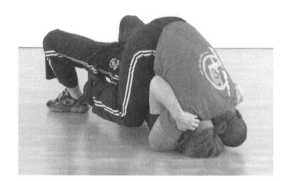

1–3. As the attacker comes in close to put his weight on you, trap the arm that is making the hold and the leg on the same side. Buck your hips upward and, at the top of the arch, roll your hips toward the trapping side. You will likely end up in his guard. If he is still holding you, push the blade of your forearm across his face (a "crossface") to force him to let go, then continue with counterattacks.

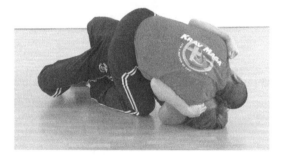

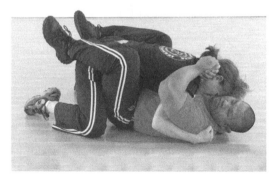

4–6. Strike immediately, if possible. However, because you're being held in so tight, it may be difficult to strike. Scratch and claw at the face, or push your forearm across his jaw (a "cross-face") to cause him to let go.

7. From here, apply initial techniques to remove yourself from the guard.]

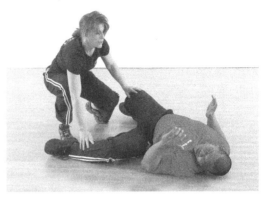

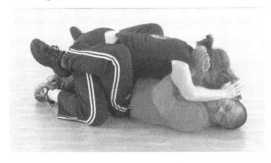

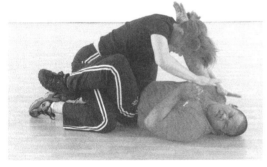

TIPS

If the attacker has you in a close choke, trap the arm on the same side that the head is positioned.

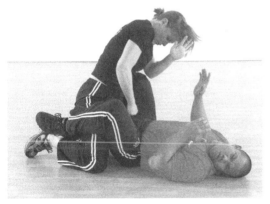

Groundfighting

An alternative to the buck-and-roll technique is the elbow escape. This technique is a bit more dangerous than the buck and roll because your hands are occupied for a longer period of time and are therefore not able to protect your face. However, against bigger or more experienced attackers, the elbow escape is more effective than the buck and roll.

STARTING POSITION: On the ground, with an attacker straddling you.

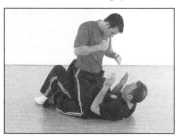

1. Wedge your left elbow between the ground and the attacker's right knee to create space. Turn onto your left hip.

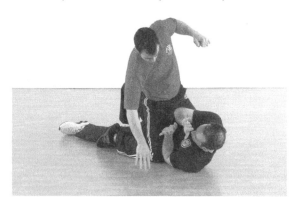

2–3. With your left leg extended and flat on the floor and the right foot flat on the floor, push ("shrimp") your hips to the right side. Use your abs to help pull your hips up and out. Your right hand can assist by helping push the attacker's right knee away.

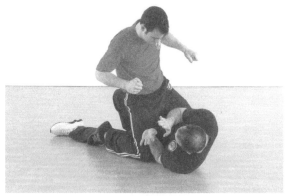

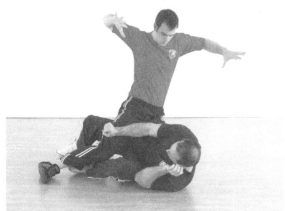

4–5. Slide your left leg under the attacker's right leg. Be sure to keep your left leg flat to avoid getting caught on the attacker's leg. Immediately use that leg to trap the attacker's leg, then shrimp in the other direction to slide the right leg under the attacker's left leg. Again, use both hands to push the attacker's knee and to create space.

6–7. Once both legs are out, pull the attacker into your guard.

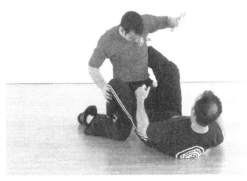

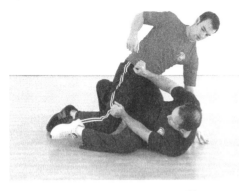

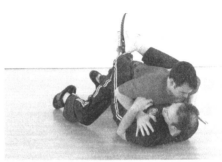

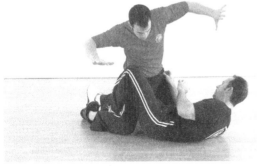

VARIATION: You can also use the elbow escape when the attacker is sitting up and leaning back in the mount position. In this situation, use your right hand (straight arm) to push at the attacker's midsection.

Simultaneously push your hip back and away aggressively, sliding your legs under the attacker's. You can either pull the attacker into the guard or continue to kick away and get up.

Groundfighting

In a fight, you may end up in a dominant position. In this section, we will discuss how to operate in this advantageous position.

MAINTAINING MOUNT

POSITION 1: When in top position of the mount, you want to maintain a good base. You do this by staying close to the defender. Keep your hips back toward your heels, knees in tight or wide to base (depending on the opponent's movement), and arms posted wide. If the defender grabs your arms, you want to pull them back quickly, bringing your elbow to your hip ("swim out"), and then re-post.

You must be able to feel the defender's weight shift and adjust to it.

You can also maintain the mount position while sitting up and back. If you stay over the defender's hips, you can keep from being bucked. However, your striking will not be strong (or may not reach) until you put your weight forward.

POSITION 2: An option is to try to move up on the defender's chest with your knees under his arms. In this position it is hard for the bottom person to defend against strikes to the face.

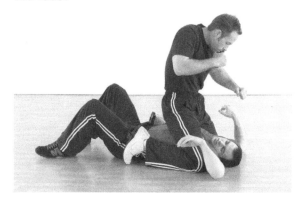

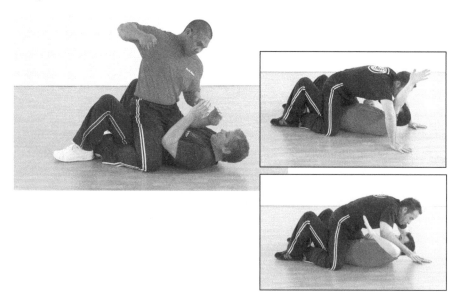

STRIKES

POSITION 3: With your hands posted and your weight low on the defender, you can send strikes to the defender's head and body. Palm strikes, elbows, and headbutts work best from this position. Be sure to always recover to your base position.

POSITIONS 4-5: For stronger strikes, sit up and back and then come down with punches and elbows.

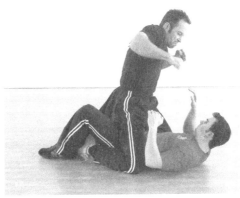

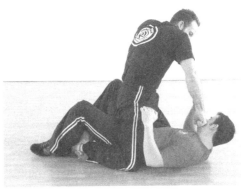

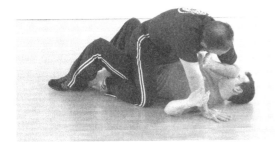

Groundfighting

Although the mount is a good position in a fight, you may need to get up from the ground to defend against a third party, or to simply disengage from the fight.

Starting Position: Mounted on top of a prone defender.

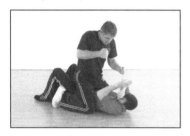

1. While sitting up and back, pin your opponent's arms to his chest—use your body weight, not just your arm strength.

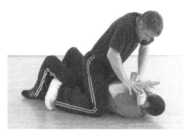

2. Pop your hips up, keeping your feet on the ground on either side of the attacker; your hands should still pin his arms.

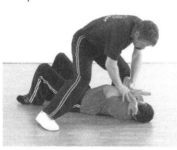

3. Lift one leg up and over, pivoting to one side of his body near his head. (Be sure to lift your leg high enough to pass over his bent knee).

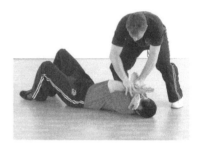

4. Stand straight up, moving away from the attacker.

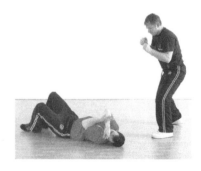

This technique presents a basic method of making distance when you've trapped someone in your guard. Additional techniques, including arm bars, will be taught at higher levels. This technique can be performed most easily when the opponent's weight is back, although it can be done when his weight is forward (it's just more difficult).

STARTING POSITION: Holding an attacker in your guard.

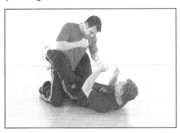

1. Shift to one hip, bringing your top knee in against his body. Your hands should be up to protect against punches.

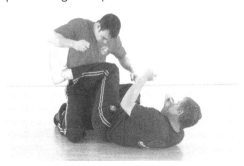

2. Kick your bottom foot against his hip to create space.

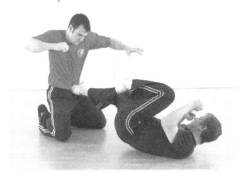

3. Kick your top foot against his chest or face.

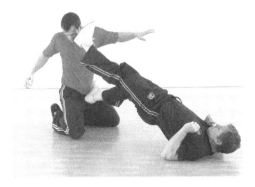

Get up and create distance.

FOOT GRAB: STRIPPING

Groundfighting

This technique can be applied when a standing attacker grabs the defender's foot.

STARTING POSITION: The defender is lying on her back. The attacker is standing up, grabbing the defender's foot.

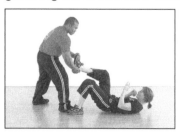

1. When the attacker grabs one of your feet, you want to remove at least one of his hands to keep him from spinning you. So raise your free foot high. At the same time, "flex" your caught leg—this gives you extra power and also helps you target his hands.

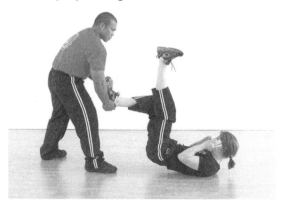

2–3. Bring your raised leg down, heel first, to strike his hand and strip it from your foot. Immediately kick at his legs to cause damage.

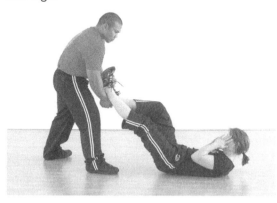

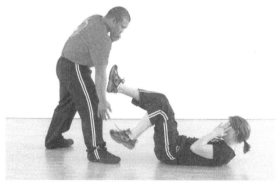

This technique is used when the attacker succeeds in catching the defender's foot and twists it outward.

STARTING POSITION:
The defender is lying on her back. The attacker is standing up, grabbing the defender's foot.

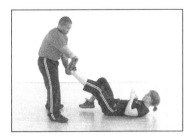

1–2. When you feel the attacker spin you, go with the motion. Do NOT resist it. Instead, spin faster than the attacker's movement. At the same time, throw a round kick in the general vicinity of his wrists.

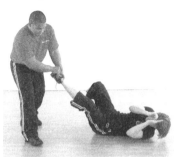

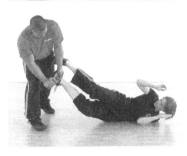

3–4. Spin through, and end up in a groundfighting position.

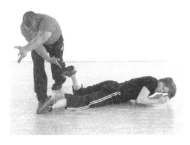

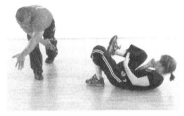

TIPS

The spin will do most of the work for you. The kick is simply insurance. The kick may also be delivered to the face if the attacker is close enough.

Groundfighting

STARTING POSITION: The defender is lying on her back. The attacker is standing up, grabbing the defender's foot.

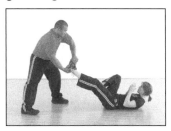

1–2. When you feel the attacker spin you, go with the motion; do NOT resist it. Instead, spin faster than the attacker's movement. At the same time, bring your leg around in a chopping/swinging motion, leading with your heel. Although the angle is different, the motion is exactly like the motion made to strip the hand off your ankle in an earlier technique.

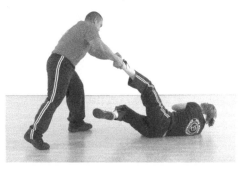

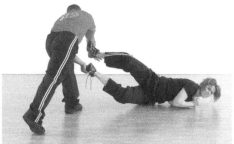

3. Continue spinning through and end up in a grounding position.

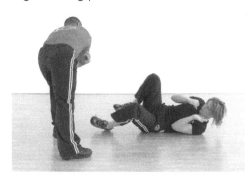

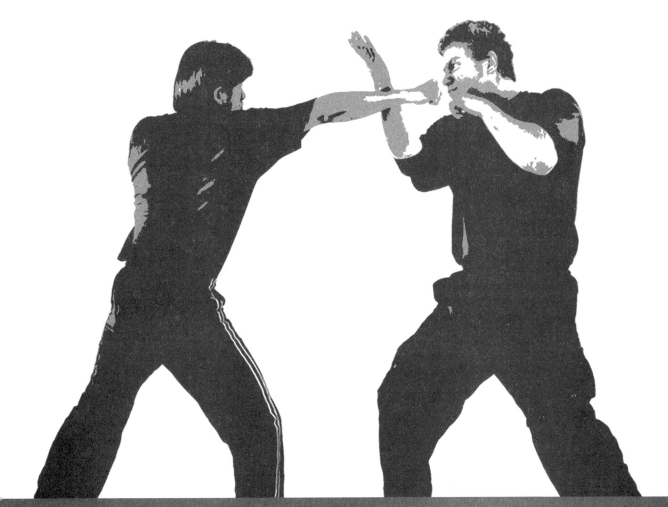

GREEN BELT

GREEN BELT

OVERVIEW

For us, Green Belt represents the beginning of real mastery of the system. When we test people for advancement to the next belt level, Green Belt is where people start to fail. It is certainly possible to fail a Yellow or Orange Belt test, but as long as the students can fight through the stress, show aggressiveness, and perform techniques adequately, they should pass Yellow and Orange.

Green Belt is where you need to bring it all together: You must deal with the stress, be aggressive, AND execute techniques sharply and cleanly. Expect to train for at least nine months at this level, assuming a minimum of two training sessions a week.

The material in this section includes the following:

COMBATIVES

Among the combative techniques covered in this section are headbutts. Green Belt also introduces more traditional martial arts kicks such as slap kick and heel kick. Although we don't stress these kicks nor emphasize them for street situations, we do believe these techniques improve our self-defense abilities. The kicks encourage flexibility as well as help us learn to defend against these types of attacks. Also, while you should always stick with the simplest and most powerful strikes, these kicks will help you feel that you can at least deliver some kind of attack from any angle during the fight.

DEFENSES AND SELF-DEFENSE

Hair grab defenses are introduced at this level, and Inside and Outside Defenses are featured more fully here. Outside Defenses against Punches are made against attacks coming from outside our hand position. Although wide attacks (such as the attacks given in 360° Defenses) and even short attacks that travel from the outside inward (such as hook punches) are common attacks to defend, they are not the only ones.

Sometimes the defender's hands are out of position (for example, the left hand is down) when a straight-line attack approaches. If your hands were up, you'd give a regular Inside Defense. But if your hands are down, the most efficient way to defend is to move your hand from the center of your body toward the outside (hence the name). Also, even if your hands were up, sometimes a straight-line attack can come in from an angle (for example, a straight punch coming in from the side), making an Inside Defense difficult. In this case, the shortest movement is an Outside Defense. This section covers both situations: 1) the defender's hands are down, due to error or fatigue; and 2) the attack comes from an angle outside the defender's correctly positioned hands. In either case, the principle behind the techniques (indeed, all the techniques) can be summarized this way: Make the shortest possible movement that defends the attack.

FALLS AND ROLLS

Rolls are important for an overall understanding of self-defense scenarios. During combat, while retreating from a fight or while advancing to help a third party, the defender may trip over an obstacle or be tripped by an opponent. Because we want to get off the ground as quickly as possible, a roll offers the most immediate solution when there is no immediate danger to address.

GROUNDFIGHTING

This section picks up where Orange Belt left off. Here you'll increase the number of techniques in your groundfighting repertoire.

FORWARD HEADBUTT

Combatives

This strike is delivered to a close target directly in front of you, such as an opponent when both of you are standing; or during grappling.

STARTING POSITION: Stand facing your opponent, nearly chest to chest. Grab your opponent's head, either by the ears or sides of the hair, for extra control and power.

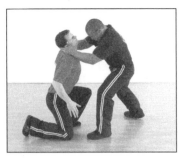

1. Keeping your neck stiff and your jaw tightly closed, drive your head forward using your legs and upper body. The striking surface is the top of your forehead, right at the hairline. The target should be the attacker's nose, cheekbone, etc

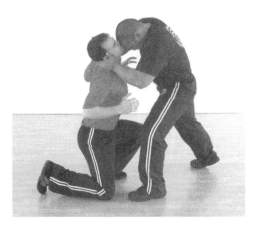

TIPS

The target should always be somewhere below the opponent's eyebrows, preferably the nose. It's not necessary to grab your opponent's head. If you do grab the head, be sure to lift his chin slightly; do not pull his chin down. If you do, you make strike his skull and injure yourself.

This can be used when you shoot in unsuccessfully on your opponent and want to drive upward to catch his chin.

STARTING POSITION: Stand facing your opponent. Duck down so that your head is at his chest level.

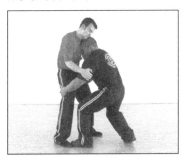

1. Keeping your neck fairly stiff and your jaw tightly closed, drive your head upward, striking with the top/back part of your skull, striking your opponent's chin.

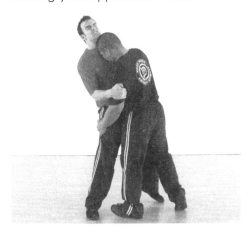

HEADBUTT TO THE SIDE

Combatives

This can be used when you're grabbed in a bearhug or any other close-in situation where your head is sideways to your attacker's face.

STARTING POSITION: Stand with your opponent close to your side, as if he is about to put you in a bearhug.

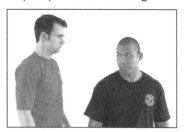

1. Turn your head sharply so that your forehead faces the target.

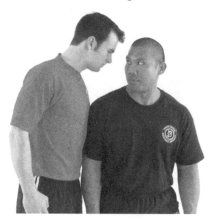

2. Keeping your neck fairly stiff and your jaw tightly closed, drive your head forward using your legs and upper body, striking with your forehead. Because of the angle, you may strike near the side of your forehead. However, do not strike with the side of your head. This may injure you.

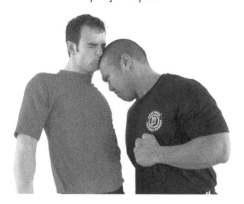

This strike is most often delivered in the context of bearhugs. It can be delivered to someone grabbing from behind, or to someone facing you when you are doubled over (in a position similar, say, to reverse headlock), when the headbutt is driven upward, but using the back of the head.

STARTING POSITION: Stand facing away from your opponent, who has you in a bearhug.

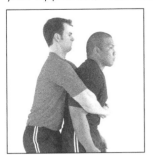

1. Send your head back sharply, flexing your neck muscles and tightening your jaw, to strike with the back of your head (near the top).

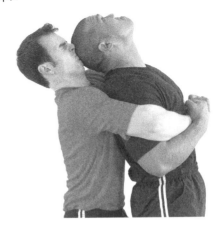

DEFENSIVE BACK KICK WITH A SPIN

Combatives

Krav Maga training de-emphasizes complicated kicks. However, of the "fancier" techniques, spinning back kick is the most practical because the direction of the kick opposes any forward motion of an attacker.

STARTING POSITION: Left-leg-forward fighting stance, facing an opponent.

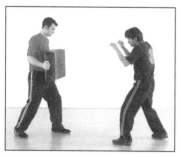

1. Step your left foot across and forward slightly. Turn sharply so that the heel of your forward (base) foot is pointing at the target. Your back is also to the target, but turn your head so that you can see the target. You should be in the same position as a regular Back Kick (page 100).

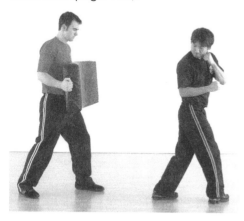

2. Extend your right leg back to make a back kick.

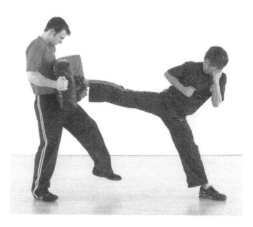

As you recoil, turn to face the target.

TIPS

Spinning kicks are always made using the rear leg.

The first step can be removed as you become more proficient, but it ALWAYS facilitates the turn.

Offensive back kick is delivered to a target behind the defender when the opening is on a horizontal plane (e.g., the groin, or the head/chest when the attacker's body is leaning forward).

STARTING POSITION: Neutral stance, with an opponent behind you.

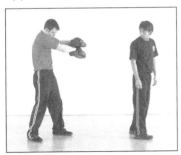

1. Raise your right leg backward, making sure it is relatively straight. At the same time, drop your body forward and swing your hips back so that your weight goes into the kick. Be sure your kicking foot rises straight up. Just before contact, bend your knee to add extra power to the kick and protect your knee from hyperextension.

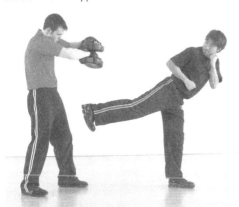

2. Make contact with the back of the heel.

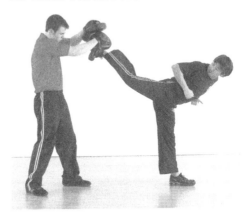

As you recoil, turn to face the attacker.

TIPS

If training from a fighting stance, the leg farthest from the target will be the strongest.

OFFENSIVE BACK KICK WITH A SPIN

Combatives

This kick simply combines an Offensive Back Kick (page 163) with the act of spinning. The kick is made with the rear foot (i.e., the foot farthest from the target before the technique begins).

STARTING POSITION: Left-leg-forward fighting stance, facing your attacker.

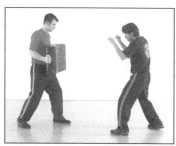

1. Take a small step across and forward with your left foot. Turn sharply so that the heel of your left (base) foot and your back are square to the target.

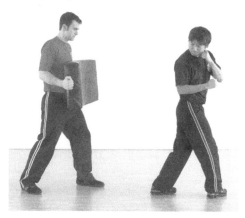

2. Raise your right leg backward, making sure it is relatively straight. At the same time, drop your body forward and swing your hips back so that your weight goes into the kick. Be sure your kicking foot rises straight up. Just before contact, bend your knee, adding extra power to the kick and protecting your knee from hyperextension.

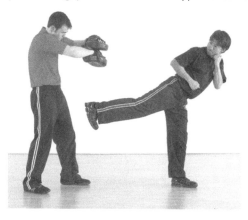

3. Make contact with the back of the heel.

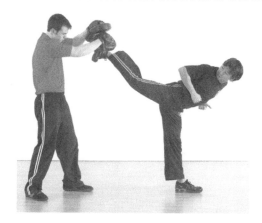

As you recoil, turn to face the attacker.

Heel kick can be made when the defender is sideways to the target, but when the opening is not on an angle appropriate to a Side Kick (page 98). The kick may be made on a rising diagonal or on a horizontal plane, depending on the opening.

STARTING POSITION: Stand sideways to your target.

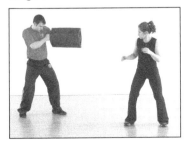

1. Raise your close leg slightly in front of the target, making sure your leg is relatively straight. As your foot rises, bend your torso over your outside hip. This will allow your leg to rise as high as necessary.

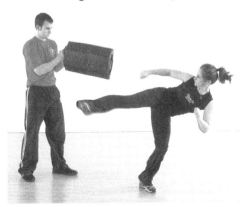

2–3. Swing you leg back, heel first, toward the target. Be sure your hip and shoulder turn in the same direction your leg is traveling. Just before contact, bend your knee, adding power to the kick and protecting the knee from hyperextension. Make contact with the back of the heel.

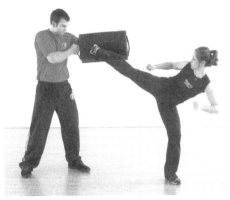

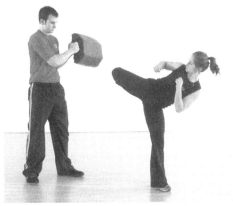

As you recoil, turn to face the attacker.

VARIATION: This kick can be made with an advance similar to Side Kick with Advance (page 99), with the base foot passing behind the kicking foot.

INSIDE SLAP KICK

Combatives

This kick is made with the inner part of the foot and ankle and attacks openings similar to those available to Round Kicks (page 47). The kick can be performed with either leg.

STARTING POSITION: Left-leg-forward fighting stance, facing your attacker.

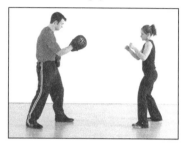

1. Raise your right knee up and forward. Emphasize "chambering" your knee to make sure it's bent.

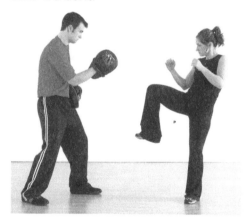

2. Leading with your knee, cant slightly inward with the foot slightly outward and snap your foot out so that it strikes the target at an approximate 45° angle. The striking point is the "L" shape of the inside of your foot and ankle.

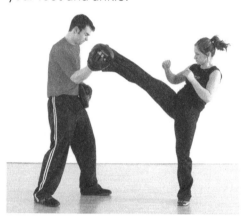

TIPS

Your hips do not roll over the way they do on a round kick.

This kick is made with the outer part of the foot and ankle and attacks openings similar to those available to Heel Kicks (page 165). The kick can be performed with either leg, but for demonstration purposes this description assumes you are kicking with the left leg.

STARTING POSITION: Left-foot-forward fighting stance, facing your attacker.

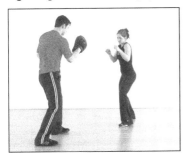

1. Bring your left knee up and across your body. Your knee should be canted slightly outward, with your foot slightly inward toward your body

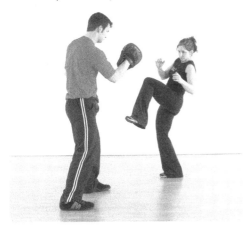

2. Snap your foot out, striking the target at an approximate 45° angle. The striking surface is the "L" shape of the outer part of your foot and ankle. Be sure your hips open up, allowing more power to transfer through the target.

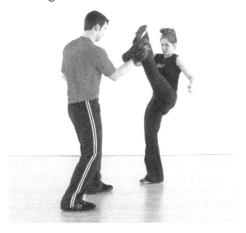

TIPS

While the forward leg delivers a faster kick, the rear leg is stronger but more easily seen because the rear hip must travel forward.

VARIATION: This kick can be made with an advance similar to Side Kick with Advance (page 99), with the base foot passing behind the kicking foot.

INWARD ANGLE KNEE

Combatives

An inward knee (familiar to Muay Thai fighters) allows the knee to be brought up and then in. It is given in a clinch, when the defender must create room to deliver the strike.

STARTING POSITION: Begin in a clinch with an opponent.

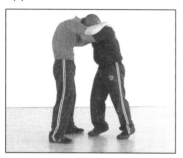

1. Lift one knee out to the side, pointing your knee toward the ceiling and your foot toward the floor.

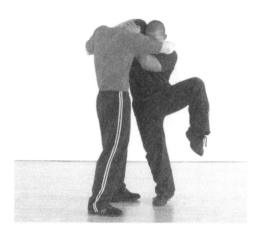

2. Drive your knee forward into the attacker, tipping your knee sharply so that it leads the motion and adds more impact on delivery.

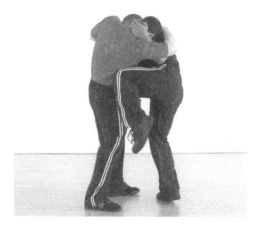

A left-right punching combination is one of the most common moves in fighting. Students should train to be aware of it and defend it.

STARTING POSITION: Left-leg-forward fighting stance, facing your attacker.

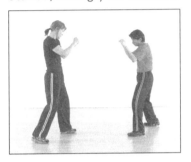

1. As your attacker throws a left punch, make an Inside Defense (page 54) with your right hand. Your left hand should be up, ready to defend against the imminent right punch.

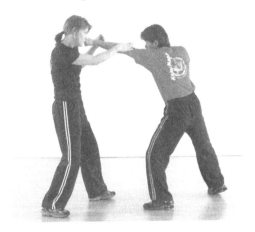

2. As your attacker throws the right punch, make an Inside Defense against it with your left hand while shifting your head to the opposite side in a body defense.

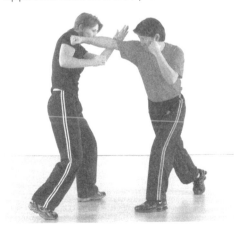

Defenses

The left-right punching combination is so common that fighters will often employ it over and over again, creating a rhythm of which they are unaware. Good fighters should notice and exploit this. The punch can be presented in two scenarios: either when the defender is surprised by the attack, or the defender sets up the attacker. Since setting up the attacker is the easier version, we'll deal with the scenario of complete surprise first.

STARTING POSITION: Left-leg-forward fighting stance, facing an opponent.

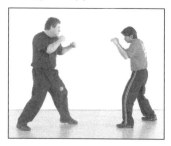

1. As the left punch comes, lean away from your attacker to avoid the left punch.

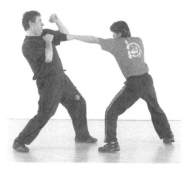

2–3. As the right punch comes, make an Inside Defense with your left hand. As soon as the defense is made, hook your left hand to clear the punching hand and counterattack. Burst in as much as possible.

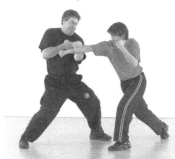

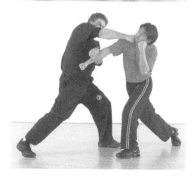

TIPS

Lean back as much as possible but make sure your feet are stable enough to allow you to burst back into the fight (your ability to do this, however, will depend on your state of readiness, and you may not be able to shift your weight much). To achieve this, stand on the ball of your back foot.

When training to "time" the opponent's punch, this technique can be very effective. Lean back as though leaving the fight. This will often make the attacker come after you, committing strongly to his right punch and leaving him open, since you are anticipating that punch. You should only attempt this technique (leaning out of the fight to sucker the attacker in) only if you've noticed a constant habit of left-right punches. Even so, always be aware that a fight can change, and the attacker may choose that moment to make a variation.

For various reasons (mainly due to injury), we may be forced to defend a left-right punching combination using only the forward hand. We never choose to defend this way.

STARTING POSITION: Left-leg-forward fighting stance, facing your attacker.

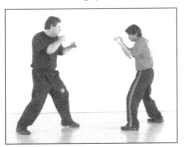

1. As the attacker throws the left punch, make an Inside Defense using your left (forward) hand.

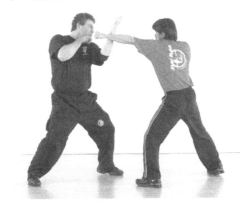

2. As the right punch comes in, immediately make an Outside Defense #1 (page 172) with the same hand, creating a chopping motion against the incoming arm.

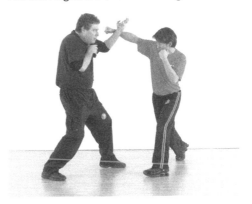

VARIATION: Using Outside Defense #3 (page 174) is possible and often safer, as it covers more variations of the straight punch.

Defenses

This defense, which redirects the attack, is made against a straight punch coming from the front when the defender's forward hand is down. Most students find this to be the quickest motion.

STARTING POSITION: Left-leg-forward fighting stance, left hand dropped forward and down, facing your attacker.

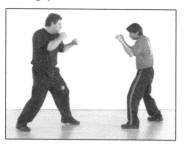

1. As the attacker throws a left punch, bring your forward hand up in a short arc, with the thumb leading so that your palm faces you. The motion of this arc MUST cross in front of your face since that's where the punch is probably going. Redirect the punch away from you while making a small body defense with your head.

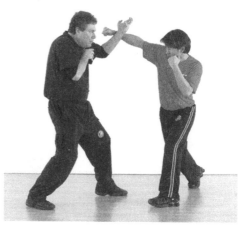

This defense, which redirects the attack, is made from the same position and against the same attack as Outside Defense #1. Most students find this defense slightly stronger than Defense #1. The decision to make Defense #1 or Defense #2 is largely arbitrary, depending on the individual's body type. However, Defense #1 is faster, while Defense #2 is stronger.

STARTING POSITION: Left-leg-forward fighting stance, left hand dropped forward and down, facing your attacker.

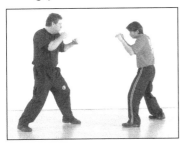

1. As the attacker throws a left punch, bring your forward hand up in a short arc, with the back of your hand leading so that your thumb faces you. The motion of this arc MUST cross in front of your face since that's where the punch is probably going. Redirect the punch away from you while making a small body defense with your head.

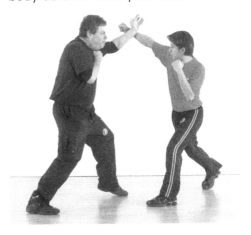

OUTSIDE DEFENSE #3

Defenses

This defense may be made against a straight punch coming from the front or the side, especially a punch coming to the head, in which case the shortest line off the body is up. This defense redirects the attack.

STARTING POSITION: Left-leg-forward fighting stance, both hands out of position, facing your attacker.

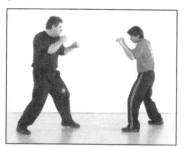

1–2. As the attacker throws a right punch toward your face, roll your left forearm up. Make contact with the blade of your arm, then continue to roll, allowing the punch to slide up and back. At the same time that you move the attacking arm, drop your head down and counterattack to the body.

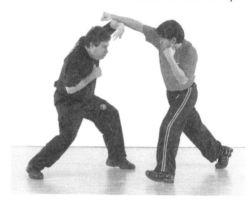

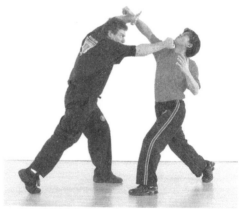

TIPS

When your head drops down, be sure that your weight doesn't drop down into your feet, making you stick in place.

Defenses

This defense is made against wild haymaker-type punches in which the defender isn't sure if the attack is coming from the inside or outside.

STARTING POSITION: Left-leg-forward fighting stance, facing your attacker.

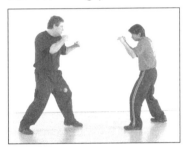

1. As the attacker throws a right punch, stab your left hand forward and slightly inward to guarantee contact. Tuck your head low, keeping your chin down but eyes forward.

2. As soon as you feel contact with your left hand, move that forearm slightly outward to increase the redirection of the punch. Allow the punch to slide along your forearm.

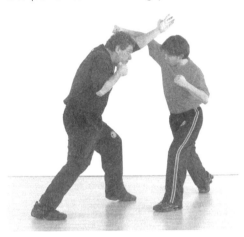

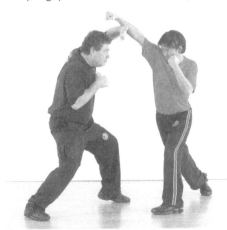

Defenses

This defense, which redirects the attack, is very similar to #1 and #2. However, the defense is made with the blade (pinky side) of the hand and arm, usually against a straight punch coming in from the side. The hands may be up or down, and even if the hands are up, this defense will be necessary against a straight punch from the side.

Starting Position: Left-leg-forward fighting stance, with your attacker at your left side, facing you.

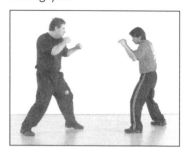

1. As the attacker throws a right punch, move your left hand in an arc to the side and forward, making contact as close to the attacker's wrist as possible to redirect the hand. As your hand rotates, allow your shoulder to open to aid in the defense and to prepare for counters. Make a body defense by taking your head inward, along the line of the defense. This will help take your head off-line if the initial punch is followed by another with the attacker's other hand.

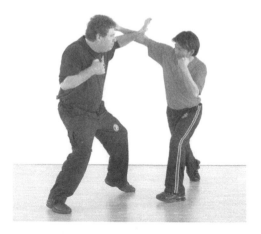

TIPS

The farther up the arm you are when you first make contact with the attacking arm, the later your defense has been.

When a right punch (or a cross coming against your jab) comes from outside your forward hand, you can defend and counter simultaneously with that hand.

STARTING POSITION: Left-leg-forward fighting stance, facing your attacker.

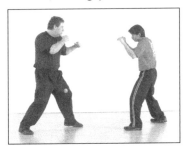

1. As the attacker throws a right punch, punch with your left hand, letting your elbow roll up in a bent position as it brushes against the attacker's punch. This diverts the attacker's punch up and away from your face.

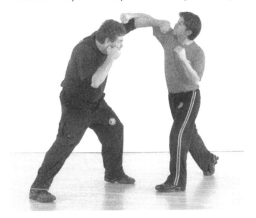

2. Continue the motion, bringing your punch down on the attacker's face.

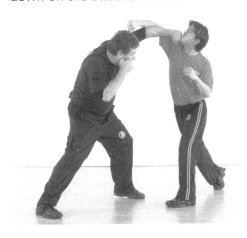

TIPS
Tuck your head in against your shoulder for additional protection.

Defenses

This defense assumes the defender is totally unprepared for the attack, which comes high to the upper torso or head.

STARTING POSITION: Neutral stance, facing your attacker.

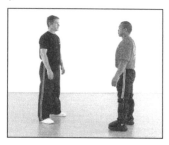

1. As the attacker begins kicking with his right leg, raise your hands defensively and turn your body so that your shoulders are square to the kick and both hands can catch the incoming leg. Your palms should be open and facing the incoming kick. Block the kick with the fleshy part of your forearms, making sure that there is enough tension in your arms to both withstand the kick and absorb the shock. Keep your chin down!

2. Immediately after defending, step diagonally forward and make counterattacks (e.g., a hammerfist with the closest hand, followed by a straight punch, or a straight punch with the rear hand).

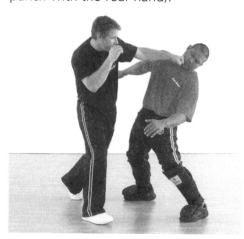

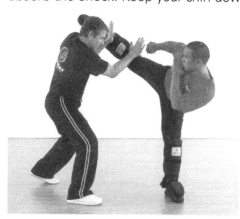

VARIATION: The defense can also be made with a diagonal step forward as you defend (to the opposite side of the kick), but this requires earlier recognition of the kick.

STARTING POSITION: Left-leg-forward fighting stance, facing your attacker.

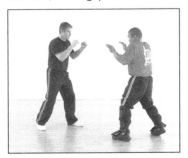

1. As the attacker begins kicking with his right leg, turn your shoulders so that they are relatively square to the kick; make a defense with your rear hand, similar to the defense against a hook punch (page 109), with your fist closed and your arm strong. At the same time, bring your opposite hand across, defending with your palm (the shoulder turn facilitates this motion).

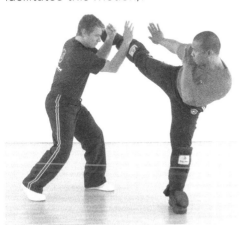

2. Follow up with counters (e.g., a hammerfist with the closest hand, followed by a straight punch, or a straight punch with the rear hand).

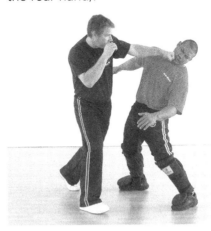

TIPS

If you prefer, you can use the reflexive version of this defense (page 178) even from a fighting stance. The reflexive defense, with the fleshy part of the forearm, provides more cushion. However, it is sometimes more difficult to rotate the forward arm around because the nature of the fighting stance inhibits the turning motion of the hips and shoulders.

Defenses

A kick defense can be made with three contact points by eliminating the shoulder rotation. Three contact points disperse the force over more area and can provide a more comfortable defense if the attacker is much bigger than you.

STARTING POSITION: Left-leg-forward fighting stance, facing your attacker.

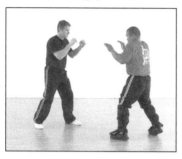

1. As the attacker begins kicking with his right leg, tuck your chin and raise your left hand parallel with your shoulder. At the same time, bring your right hand across to defend with your palm; this hand should line up with your shoulder and left hand.

Follow up with counters (e.g., a hammerfist with the closest hand, followed by a straight punch, or a straight punch with the rear hand).

TIPS

When making this defense, you MUST tuck your chin and try to cover your head. Although this kick disperses more force, it allows the kick to come much closer to your head and you may be open to kicks with the toe (booted feet) or the ball of the foot.

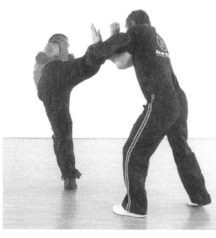

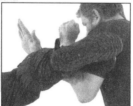

Sometimes the defender does not recognize the kick in time to make a two-handed defense. In this case, the only choice is to make a covering defense. This defense is essentially the same as a hook punch defense (page 109) but with a closed fist, combined with a body defense if time allows.

STARTING POSITION: Left-leg-forward fighting stance, facing your attacker.

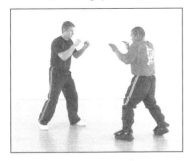

1. As the attacker begins kicking with his right leg, make a tight 360°-type defense with your left hand. Your defense should be made with a tight fist, and your forearm should be angled slightly inward so that rising kicks may slide up the arm, reducing the impact against the forearm. At the same time, step diagonally forward, away from the power of the kick.

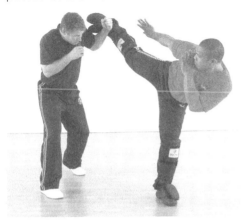

2. Counterattack with a front or round kick with the rear leg.

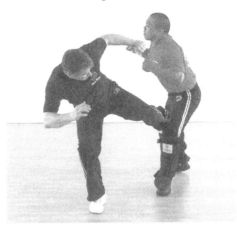

TIPS

DO NOT "reach out" to defend the kick far from your body. Your arm won't be strong at this distance and can be seriously injured by a strong kick.

Depending on how early the defender recognizes the attack, the step may not be possible. However, even if you lean or step on contact, you should move your body to get out of the kick's power zone.

Falls and Rolls

The principles of regular fall break (page 136) apply to high fall break as well, both for back falls and side falls. The only difference is in the angle your arms take as you strike the ground. With regular fall break, the angle of the slap is approximately 45° away from the body. As the angle of the fall increases (i.e., as your feet go higher into the air and your head travels more directly toward the ground), the angle of your slap should increase. During a drastic fall break, your hands go out as wide as your shoulders.

STARTING POSITION: From standing, tuck your chin to protect your neck. This protects your head and neck (and avoids the risk of biting your tongue).

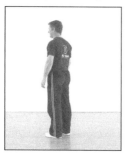

1. To imitate high fall breaks, you must throw your feet into the air so that your feet are higher than your head during the fall break.

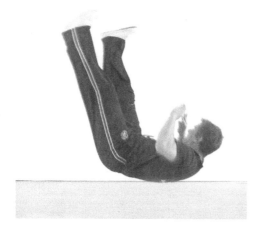

2. As you reach the ground, strike it hard with your palms at about a 90° angle. Do not lead with your elbows; if they strike the ground, you may seriously damage them.

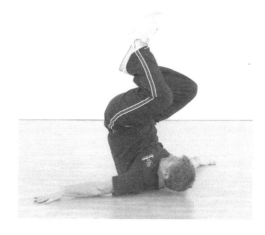

3. Immediately recoil your hands into a fighting position.

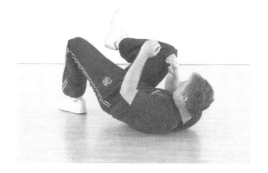

The main goal of a safe roll is to limit the amount of time spent rolling over the spine. Therefore, the roll is made on a diagonal from one shoulder to the opposite hip. This means the movement along the ground crosses the spine at only one point. These instructions assume you are right-handed. Switch "right" to "left" and vice versa if you are left-handed.

STARTING POSITION: Step forward with your right foot.

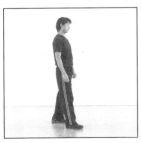

1. Bend down and place your right hand flat on the ground with your fingers pointing to the left. Place your left hand on the ground with the fingers facing forward. This position should cause your right shoulder to "lead" the motion. Tuck your chin under your left armpit (the more you tuck your chin, the safer your neck will be).

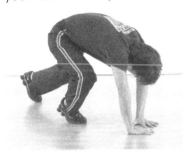

2–4. Roll over your right arm, then let the right elbow bend to roll over from your right shoulder to your left hip, leading with your right shoulder and rounding your back. As you roll, position your legs in a figure 4, with the left leg bent and the right leg relatively straight (but not completely). This figure-4 position allows you to rise into a fighting stance at the completion of the roll.

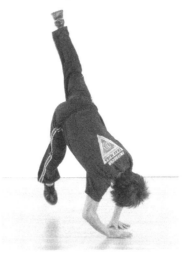

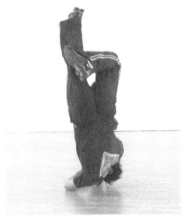

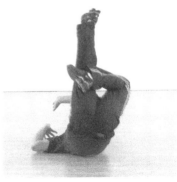

steps 5–9 continued on next page

continued from previous page

5–7. As you complete the roll, come up into a kneeling position, with your right foot and your left knee on the ground. Note that the ball of your left foot, not the top, should be touching the ground.

8–9. From this kneeling position, stand up. The foot position you've created moves you easily into a fighting stance facing the opposite direction of the roll.

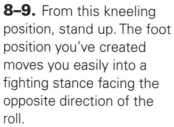

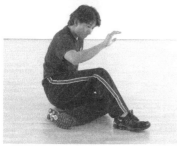

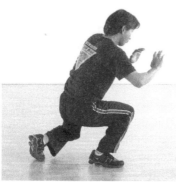

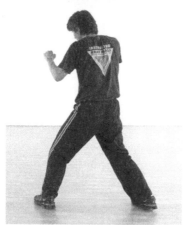

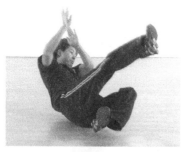

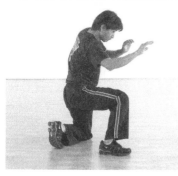

It's possible that, while running at high speed, the defender trips and makes a roll with such velocity that it's difficult to complete the roll with control. In this case, the roll is modified to include a fall break. As with the descriptions of other rolls, these instructions assume a right-handed defender leading with the right shoulder. Reverse all directions if the left shoulder leads.

STARTING POSITION: Begin at a run.

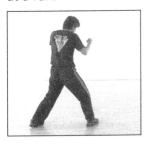

1–2. Make an initial high-speed roll, leading with your right hand and shoulder.

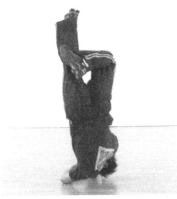

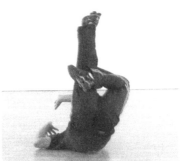

3–4. Halfway through the roll, assuming you have too much velocity (and therefore too little control) to complete the motion, make a back fall break.

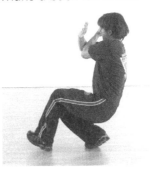

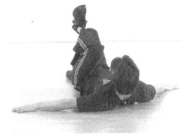

BACKWARD ROLL

Falls and Rolls

STARTING POSITION: Sitting or lying on your back.

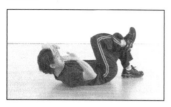

1. Roll backward toward one shoulder, sending both hands over that same shoulder. Do NOT roll straight back over your head. Be sure to tuck your chin!

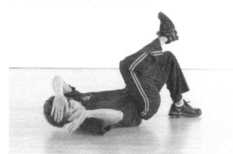

2. Bring your legs over that same shoulder.

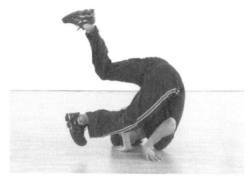

3. Roll up onto your feet into a fighting stance.

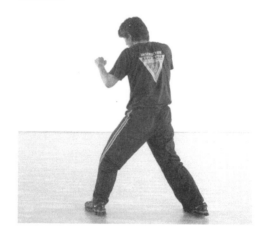

STARTING POSITION:
Attacker has you in a reverse headlock, also known as a guillotine choke.

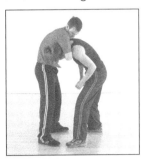

1. Turn your head toward the attacker's hands (the weakest part of the choke); make a plucking motion with your outside hand to relieve the pressure, while striking to the groin with your free hand. You can also throw up an elbow to strike the face, but the groin is the easiest target.

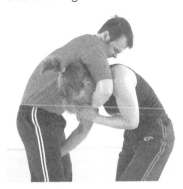

2–3. Once you pluck, drive your right shoulder into the space you have created to ensure you can no longer be choked. Drive your shoulder and head forward and upward as though trying to go through his hold; emphasize driving upward, which puts pressure on his shoulder. Your free hand may help hold his hands in place.

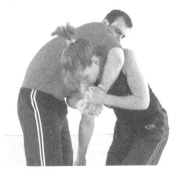

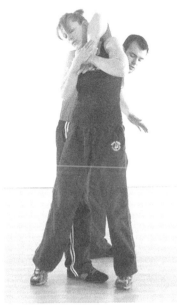

4. Once his hold is broken, spin toward him and deliver counterattacks with knees, punches, and elbows.

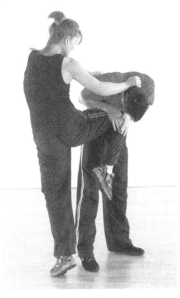

TIPS

If the attacker is very strong and determined, you may not be able to break his hold. However, if you can succeed in plucking to create space and then inserting your shoulder, he will have difficulty choking you. If you find yourself stuck here, continue with strikes and knees to the groin. Your goal is to keep his hips back so that it is harder for him to finish the choke.

HAIR GRAB FROM THE FRONT

Self-Defense

STARTING POSITION:
Attacker grabs your hair from the front.

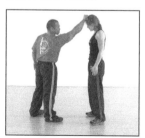

1. Bring both hands up and slam them sharply down over his hand. This punches his knuckles against your skull, causing him pain. Keep your elbows in so that your forearms protect your face against a punch (very likely combination with the hair grab).

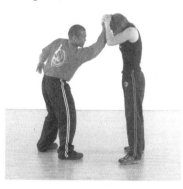

2. Immediately bend your body sharply at the waist (think of taking a bow). Bend forward to produce immediate pressure against his wrist.

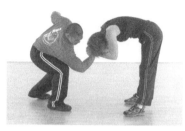

3. As the attacker drops down, quickly move backward to stretch out his body.

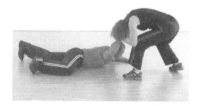

4. Immediately follow up with front kicks to the face.

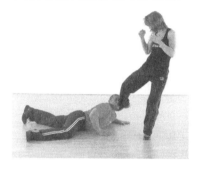

TIPS

Do not send your hips backward when you bend as this relieves the pressure in the wrist.

HAIR GRAB FROM THE FRONT OR SIDE (IMPENDING KNEE STRIKE)

If you feel yourself being pulled down by the hair grab, it's quite likely that the attacker is making a knee strike to your face. If you began to respond immediately with the regular defense against Hair Grab from the Front (page 188), continue to make it. Although this is not an optimum defense, if you have begun this motion, there will be no time to adjust. As long as your elbows are in tight, they may protect you from the knee strike.

STARTING POSITION:
Attacker grabs your hair from the side and begins to make a knee strike.

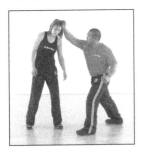

1. As your upper body is pulled down, burst inward with the pull. Make 360° Defense, position #7 (page 53) with the closest arm against the rising thigh. Be sure to block the thigh, not the knee. At the same time, strike to the groin with your free hand. It is possible that you end up "crossblocking" (i.e., you defend with your left hand against the attacker's left knee). If this is the case, your counterattack may be delayed. Make it as soon as possible after the defense.

2. Continue driving forward with your body to relieve any remaining pressure or control from the hair grab. If possible, straighten up to avoid any more knee strikes to the face, and continue with counters.

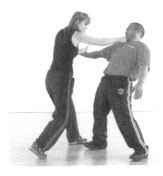

TIPS

If the hair grab is from the front and no more knee strikes are coming, you can continue with regular Hair Grab from the Front.

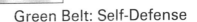

HAIR GRAB FROM THE SIDE

Self-Defense

If you feel yourself being pulled down, make the defense against Hair Grab—Impending Knee Strike (page 189). It's also possible that the attacker is simply pulling you off balance, or pulling you toward some goal (a car, an alley). In either case (a downward pull or lateral pull), one principle remains the same: You must burst in the direction of the pull at a speed faster than the pull itself. If the pull is five miles an hour, burst in at six miles an hour. Only by bursting in faster than the pull can you regain control of your body movement.

STARTING POSITION: Attacker grabs your hair from the side.

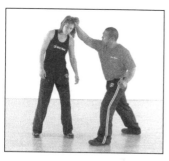

1. As the attacker pulls, do not resist. Burst in the direction of the pull, ideally toward the shoulder of the hand that is holding your hair. This limits your vulnerability to a punch from the attacker's free hand.

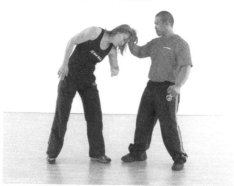

2. As you burst in, reach up with your close hand to clear the hand holding your hair.

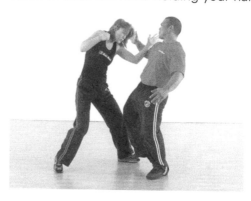

3. With your free hand, counterattack—the fastest and simplest counterattack is usually a punch to the face or groin.

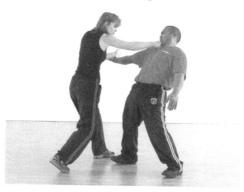

TIPS
Remember: If you feel yourself being pulled down, make a 360° Defense against the knee strike that is most likely coming.

Self-Defense

It's possible that the attacker comes from the side but grabs the hair on the back of your head, or reaches around to the other side. It's also possible that an attacker comes from the back and grabs the back of your head.

STARTING POSITION:
Attacker grabs your hair from behind.

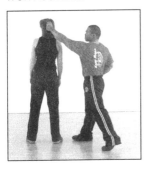

1. When you feel the pull, do not resist. Instead, burst in the direction of the pull, ideally toward the shoulder of the hand that has grabbed you. You may feel yourself "spin" around. Go with this motion (e.g., if the attacker on your left reaches around and grabs the right side of your head and pulls, you will feel yourself spinning to your right. Go in that direction).

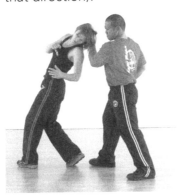

2. As you spin around, make a 360° Defense (if necessary) with the closest hand.

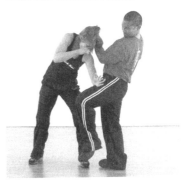

3-4. Follow up with groin and head strikes.

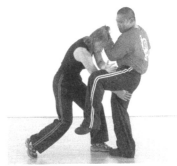

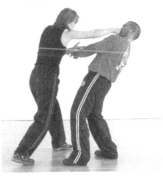

BEARHUG FROM BEHIND (LEVERAGE ON THE FINGER)

Self-Defense

When an attacker makes a bearhug from behind, leaving your arms free, he may also hide his head against your back to limit your ability to make counterattacks with your elbows. Stomps, heel strikes to his shins, and uppercut back kicks are still possible, but the attack may require another technique to remove the attacker's arms from around your body.

STARTING POSITION: Attacker bearhugs you from behind, leaving your arms free.

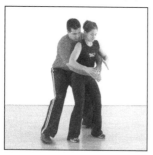

1. Immediately drop your weight to make yourself difficult to lift.

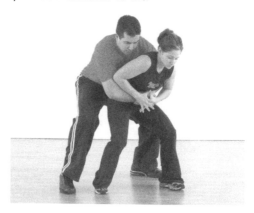

2. Make elbow strikes to the face as well as other counterattacks, such as stomps.

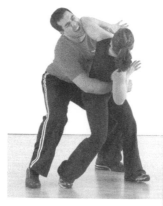
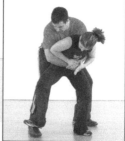

3. Slide your hands along his forearms until you find a finger (usually the index finger). Using either hand, peel the finger up, starting at the tip so that you only deal with one part of the finger at a time. If you try to pry the finger up from the base of the digit, or halfway to the tip, the attacker's grip will be too strong.

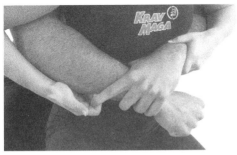

4. As you loosen the finger, begin to grab it with your opposite hand (i.e., if you get the left hand, grab the finger with your right) so that the meaty part of your hand is near the base of the finger, and the thumb side of your hand is at the tip. Think of "pushing" the finger rather than "pulling" it. Your other hand should catch the attacker's hand, isolating the finger joint. Press the finger down into its socket, then push back toward the top of the hand. This releases the bearhug.

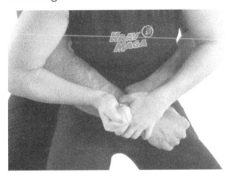

5–6. Step out, pivoting on your foot and keeping pressure on the finger.

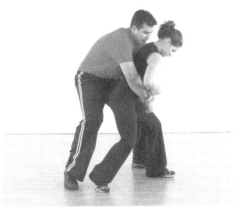

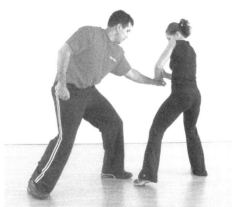

7. With your closest foot, kick to the groin or face.

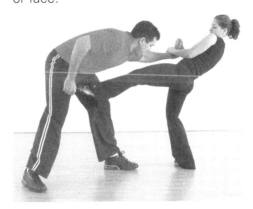

BEARHUG FROM BEHIND (WITH LIFT)

Self-Defense

STARTING POSITION: Attacker bearhugs you from behind (arms caught or arms free).

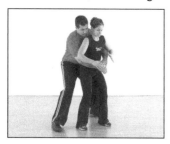

1. As the attacker lifts you, immediately make an uppercut back kick to the attacker's groin. At the same time, wrap your free leg around the attacker's leg, then straighten it as much as possible. This "wrap" limits the attacker's ability to throw you around or toss you.

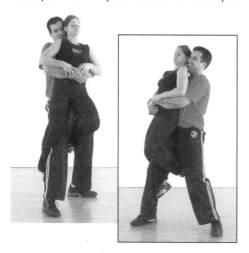

2. If you land a solid strike to the groin, the attacker will drop you quickly. Be ready to get your feet under you fast!

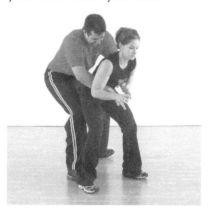

TIPS

Although the wrap is important, do NOT wait until after you've wrapped to make the kick. The kick must be immediate.

VARIATION: If you are dropped, turn and continue with counterattacks.

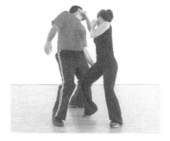

STARTING POSITION: Attacker bearhugs you from the front, encasing your arms, and lifts you.

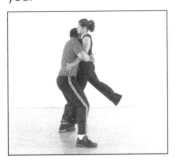

1. As the attacker lifts you, immediately make counterattacks with your knees. Knees are possible in this instance because the attacker himself becomes your base.

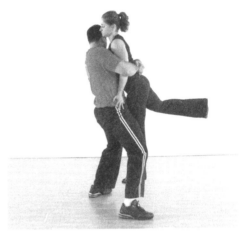

2. If you land a solid strike to the groin, the attacker will drop you quickly. Be ready to get your feet under you fast!

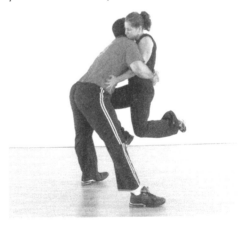

VARIATION: If your arms are free, it is also possible to grab his hair or gouge his eyes, force his chin up, and counterattack with hammerfist strikes to the face or throat in a motion similar to Bearhug from the Front with Arms Free—Leverage on the Neck (page 130).

ARM BAR FROM THE GUARD

Groundfighting

From the guard, we generally prefer to kick out and get up rather than remain on the ground and attempt grappling techniques. However, some locks, such as this one, are very practical to know. This technique is very effective if the attacker makes the mistake of straightening his arm while fighting or attempting to escape the guard. In sport fighting, this technique can cause the opponent to "tap," or surrender. When your life is threatened on the street, this technique may be used to damage or break the attacker's arm.

STARTING POSITION: On your back, holding the attacker in your guard.

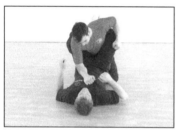

1. As the attacker straightens his arm in an attempt to escape, grab hold of his straightened arm and pull. The grab should be made with one hand on his elbow and the other hand on his wrist for the most secure hold.

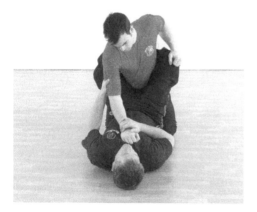

2–3. As you pull, bring your near leg up and over his head to wrap around his neck. As you do this, shift your hips so that they are perpendicular to the attacker, if possible. Keep pulling to make sure your hips and groin get close to his shoulder. This ensures that his elbow will be above the line of your groin.

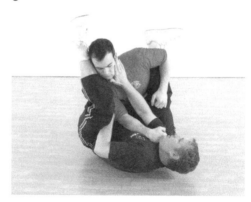

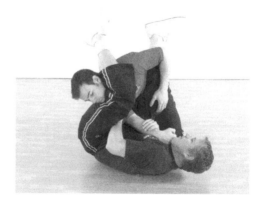

4–5. If possible, use the leg motion to take him down onto his back, although this action is not necessary for the exercise to be successful. If he stays upright, or even if he rolls the other way and you end up on your stomach, the arm lock can still work.

6. Squeeze your knees together, pull the pinky side of his hand to your chest, and push out with your hips. This puts pressure on his elbow. Be careful in training!

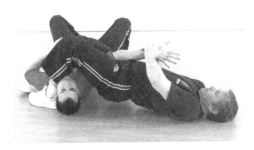

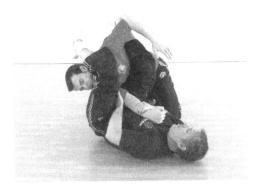

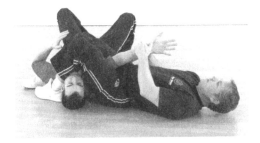

GUARD REVERSAL (SIT UP AND SWEEP)

Groundfighting

Kicking off from the guard will be your most common technique when you find yourself on your back with someone in your guard. However, some determined attackers will not allow you to create much distance or get away. In these cases, you need to know how to reverse your position, rather than just escape. This reversal can be done when the attacker, in your guard, sits back to punch.

STARTING POSITION: On your back, holding the attacker in a closed guard.

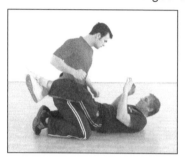

1. As the attacker sits back, sit up and put your feet on the floor.

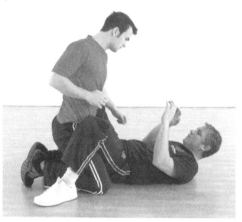

2. Post one hand (NOT your elbow) on the floor and lift your hips; reach your opposite hand up and across to the attacker's opposite side. Keep your chin down; your reach should also shield your face from punches. With your reaching hand, grab the back of his arm on or above his elbow.

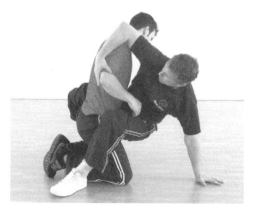

3–5. Pull his elbow/arm in and down (as though trying to pull him under you) while driving with your outside hip to help turn him over.

If you use a closed guard (ankles crossed), you'll need to release your legs before you can put your feet on the floor.

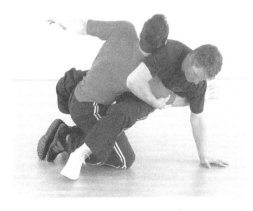

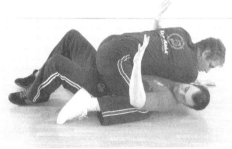

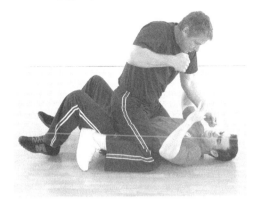

CHOKE FROM THE SIDE DEFENSE

Groundfighting

STARTING POSITION: On your back, with the attacker kneeling on your right side and applying a choke.

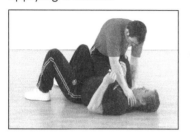

1. Make a right-handed palm heel strike to the attacker's sternum or face as you make a pluck with your left hand. The strike is made only to create space.

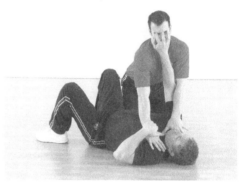

2. Immediately roll your hips up, tuck your right knee in against the attacker's chest, and bring your left foot into the air. As you tuck your right knee into the attacker's chest, bring your right hand back and grab the defender's left hand. Both your hands should now be holding and pulling on the attacker's right hand.

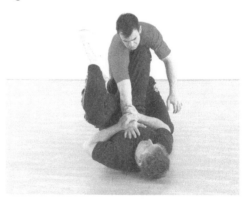

3. Bring your left leg down in a sharp motion along the left side of the attacker's neck. Your goal should be both to strike and to bring him toward the ground.

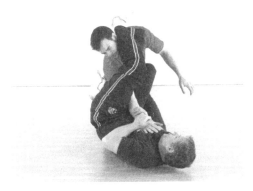

4. As you take him down, focus on bringing your left heel to your buttocks. This will keep the attacker close to you and give you more control. Continue to pull on the attacker's right arm to maintain control and keep him close.

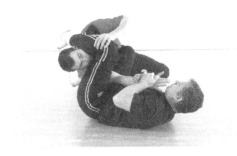

5–6. As the attacker hits the ground, bring your right foot up across his chest. If you have kept him close and pulled on the arm, the attacker's left elbow will be above the line of your groin. He is now in a position for the Arm Bar (page 196).

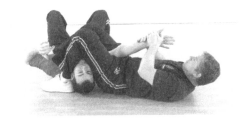

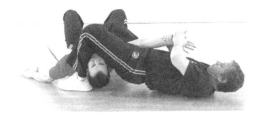

TIPS

Once you apply the arm bar, you may also continue with stomps to the attacker's face and midsection.

VARIATION: Because Krav Maga emphasizes simplicity, a less-complex version of the defense is possible. Instead of taking the attacker down with your left foot, simply "stomp" upward toward his face and kick the attacker away. If you meet resistance, you may have to perform the takedown.

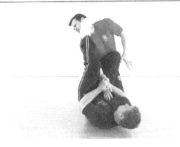

Groundfighting

This is a very common way for a groundfight to end up. Unless the attacker is much bigger and stronger, the attack offers less danger than would appear. The defender can be punched and a choke is possible, though unlikely. However, a "neck crank" is possible. There are three basic techniques with which to escape from this hold. However, two of them are very similar, and can be considered one technique. We discuss basic positioning first since the movements described in later sections all play off of this position.

THE POSITION: When the attacker applies the headlock while sitting to your right side, tuck your chin to avoid being punched or choked and shift your hips so that you are on your side.

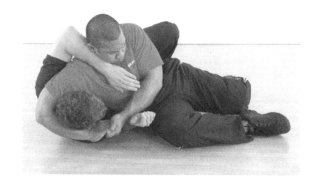

Raise your free (upper) hand up and place your forearm across your attacker's neck and jaw. This arm can be used to push against the attacker's throat/neck/head to prevent him from applying maximum pressure against your head and neck.

Tuck your other (lower) hand in. Do not let this hand get caught inside your attacker's outside hand because he will trap it there easily.

If you feel your attacker leaning forward, execute the following finishing move.

STARTING POSITION:
Headlock from the Side Defense Basic Positioning (page 202).

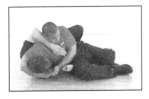

1. Reach your top leg over and hook the attacker's leg.

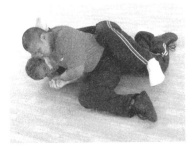

2. Pull on his leg as you straighten yours. Simultaneously use your top arm to push against his neck, and drive your top hip into his. Your weight should travel toward his head. This action should also cause your lower hip to slide out from underneath him.

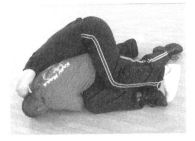

3–4. As he is forced forward, drive your shoulder downward into his, creating pressure on his arm and neck. In most cases, this will release the headlock.

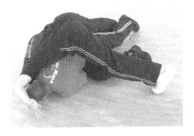

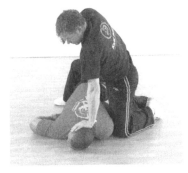

TIPS

Be sure to drive your weight toward his head, where he has no base.

VARIATION: If the attacker continues to maintain the headlock, continue to shift your hips until you are in a crouched position, on the other side of his body, with the attacker on his side beneath you. Be careful to maintain your balance. Deliver hammerfist strikes to his face, or gouge out his face and eyes.

If the headlock persists, make a palm heel strike against his jaw line, driving upward with your shoulders to stretch him out. This is called a "cross-face."

Groundfighting

Although this technique appears dissimilar from the previous exercise and will have a slightly different result, the movements made are almost exactly the same. This technique is done when a smart attacker, attempting to avoid the leg hook of the previous technique, leans forward but also scoots his legs forward to stay out of your reach. Although this makes a leg hook difficult, it creates space that you can use to your advantage.

STARTING POSITION: Headlock from the Side Defense Basic Positioning (page 202).

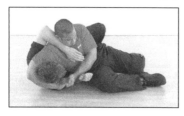

1. Reach your top leg over, as though trying to hook the attacker's leg.

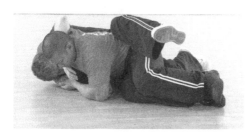

2. Failing to hook the leg, continue the motion so that your hips shift. At the same time, draw your knees up so that you are on your knees next to your attacker. Your lower hand should be ready to base out and stabilize your position. From here, the greatest danger of the headlock is essentially neutralized, although you still have a strong fight on your hands.

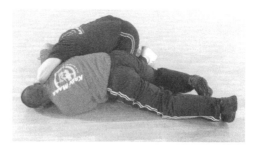

3–4. From this position, you can either slip out of the headlock, deliver counterattacks, or even make a defense against headlock from the side (page 202).

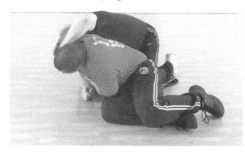

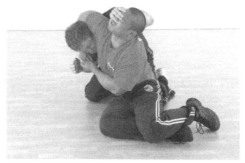

Attackers will sometimes shift their weight backward to apply more pressure to the neck or to avoid being taken forward.

STARTING POSITION: Headlock from the Side Defense Basic Positioning (page 202).

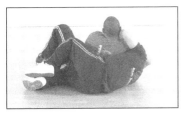

1–2. With your upper arm, push the attacker's upper body backward, toward your own hips. At the same time, quickly scoot your hips out of the way. Your hips MUST move quickly or you will stall the technique.

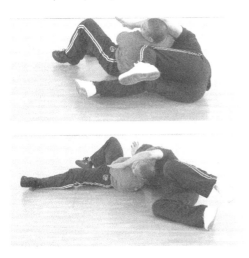

3. As the attacker rolls back, pull yourself up to your knees, making sure your bottom hand is available to base out in case he attempts to roll you.

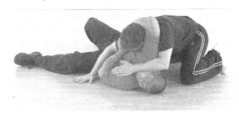

4. Attack with hammerfists, claw at the face, knees to the back, or cross-face (see note under Headlock from the Side Defense—Attacker's Weight Forward on page 203) until he releases your head.

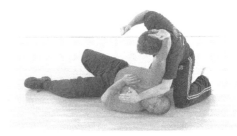

Groundfighting

STARTING POSITION: Attacker is on his back, holding you tight in his guard.

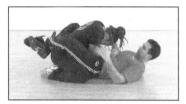

1–2. Drive forward and make constant attacks to his face with punches, hammerfists, headbutts, scratches, eye gouges, etc. Be sure to protect against arm bars by holding your elbows in tight.

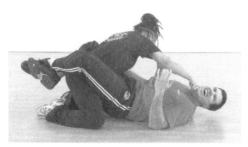

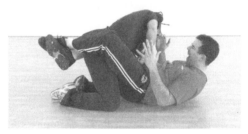

3. Drive your weight forward to "roll" or "stack" him so that his hips are higher than his head. Your hips should lie against the backs of his thighs so that he bears your weight as well as his own. Squeeze your knees against his legs. Your feet should move up and spread out to stabilize you.

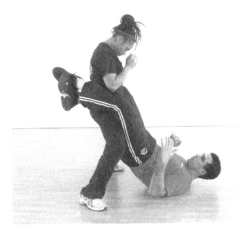

4. Deliver more counterattacks. You should be in a better position to deliver more punches.

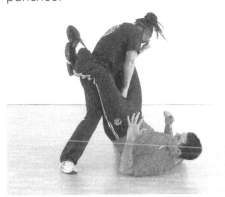

5. If he releases his guard, get up and out.

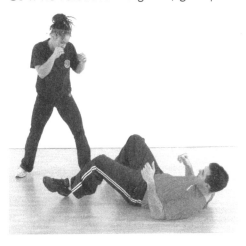

Don't lean your weight too far forward or you'll get rolled. Don't bring your feet too far forward or he'll grab them.

VARIATION: If he loosens, but does not release, his guard, try to kneel back down with your weight back. You'll still be in the guard, but you will now have space to punch to the groin.

SIDE MOUNT (BASIC POSITION)

Groundfighting

Side mount is an excellent position from the top. It's often more stable than a full mount because the attacker (on bottom) is less able to use his hips to buck you off.

THE HOLD: With the attacker on the ground, sprawl your upper body over his torso. Put your weight through your chest onto his body, keeping your elbows pressed in against his body and head to keep him tight.

Pull your bottom knee (the one closest to his hip) up so it presses tightly against his body and hip, and extend your top leg (the one closest to his head) out so that your hip touches the floor.

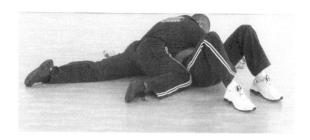

VARIATION: It is also acceptable to do a side mount by having both knees up and under you. This position allows for better striking, but removes some of the pressure from the attacker's chest, allowing him more freedom of movement. If you adopt this position, be sure that the top knee is pressed close to his upper body, and that your hands and arms are positioned to stop him from shifting his hips away to create space.

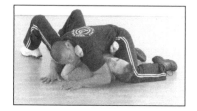

This technique is good if you feel the need to control the attacker (or, alternately, break his arm) rather than strike.

STARTING POSITION: Assume a Side Mount (page 208) on the attacker's right side so that his left arm is on the outside.

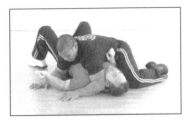

1. With your left hand, push down on the attacker's left wrist using a thumb-less grip.

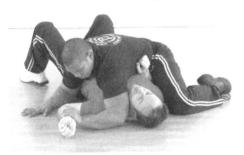

2. With the back of his hand on the floor, reach underneath his arm with your right hand and catch your own wrist—again, using the thumb-less grip. Keep your body and knee(s) close to him so that he cannot pivot away, and keep your weight on top of him. One of his defenses will be to turn his body to relieve the pressure.

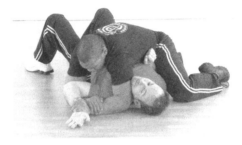

3. Keeping the back of his hand on the ground, slide his hand toward his hip. At the same time, lift your right elbow, which will crank his left elbow, causing extreme pressure on his shoulder.

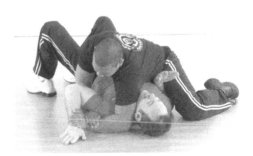

Groundfighting

In Krav Maga, from the top position we prefer to strike whenever possible since the defender can generate power and because striking generally allows the defender to disengage when he feels it is appropriate. From the side position, the primary "technique" is not the strike itself. All the strikes are basic. The main concern is that the defender learns to strike while also maintaining a solid position to prevent the attacker from gaining an advantage. The defender should practice delivering one or two strikes and then check his position. You can apply the following strikes:

STARTING POSITION: Basic Side Mount position (page 208).

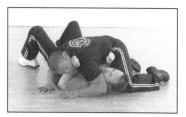

STRIKE 1: Elbow downward to the side of the attacker's head.

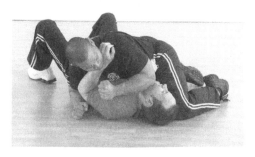

STRIKE 2: Elbow downward to the attacker's face.

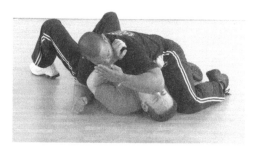

STRIKE 3: Knees to the head.

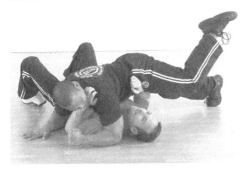

STRIKE 4: Knee to the body.

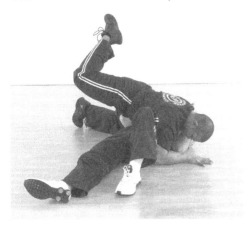

STRIKE 5: Headbutt (if safe).

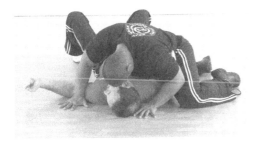

STRIKE 6: Bite.

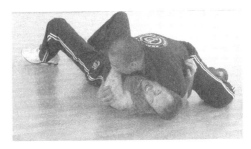

STRIKE 7: Eye gouge.

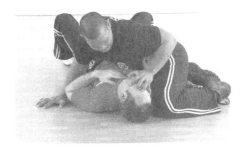

STRIKE 8: Hammerfist punches (although elbows are stronger).

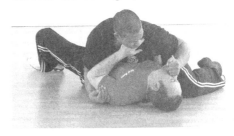

<table>
<tr><td>

TIPS
</td></tr>
</table>

Strike with either knee and either hand, but remember, he may try to change positions by shifting his hips away from you. If your lower hand is up and striking, you may give him the opening he needs to create distance.

SIDE MOUNT (TRANSITION TO FULL MOUNT)

Groundfighting

The side mount is a position of great advantage. However, the defender may feel the need or desire to transition to a full mount.

STARTING POSITION: Assume a Side Mount (page 208).

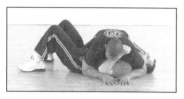

1. Slide your bottom knee (the one closest to his hip) up and across his stomach. If you lift your knee into the air, he may slip under you; if you try to move your knee across a lower part of his body, his own knee may block you.

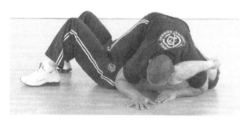

2. As your knee and leg reach the far side of his body, bring your knee to the ground.

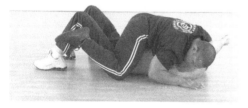

3. Bring your other leg close to him to complete the mount position.

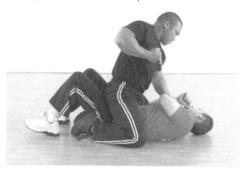

Remember, if you allow too much space to be created, you may give the attacker room to improve his position. Always stay tight!

Throughout this entire move, your goal should be to stay as high on his body (toward his chest) as possible, rather than down by his hips.

VARIATION: If he uses his knee to block your movement, push down on his knee with your lower hand.

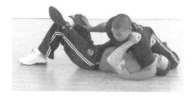

The defender should know how to safely disengage from any position, including side mount. The following technique can be used either to remain in position and continue striking, or to attack the attacker briefly and then disengage.

STARTING POSITION: Assume a Side Mount (page 208).

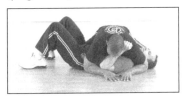

1. Slide your bottom knee (the one closest to his hip) up onto his stomach, almost as though moving into a full mount.

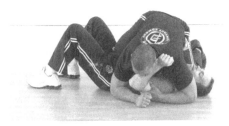

2. Press your knee and shin into his stomach and come up onto your other foot. Be sure your weight is on your knee so that he feels it!

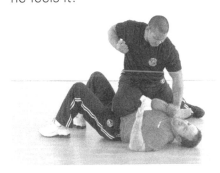

3. Continue with strikes to neutralize and/or occupy him.

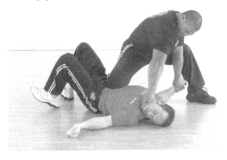

4. Step up and away, moving off quickly to avoid having your legs/feet caught.

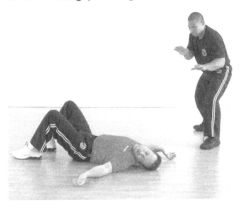

VARIATION: While striking, it may help if you can fold his arms in on themselves or otherwise trap them.

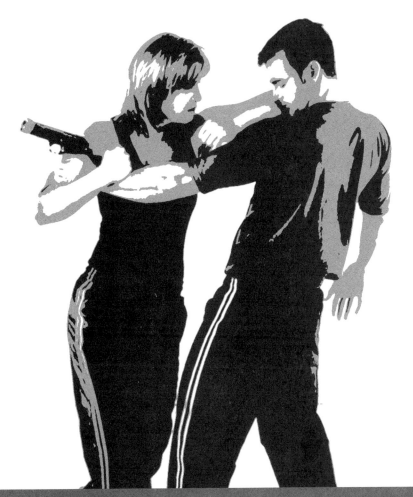

BLUE
BELT

BLUE BELT

OVERVIEW

We consider Blue Belt (sometimes called "Level 4") to be the first advanced belt in our system. At this level, your training moves beyond basic fighting skills and self-defense—you now learn to defend against threats and attacks with weapons such as guns and sticks, and you are introduced to the principles of defenses against a knife. In addition, since a Blue Belt practitioner should have solid, practical experience in fighting, fighting becomes a significant factor during the Blue Belt test.

Although we consider Blue Belt to be "advanced" training, you should keep one thing in mind: Even at high levels, our Krav Maga techniques are simple. They do, however, require aggressive and decisive action, which is why we save them for students who have learned the basic techniques and are accustomed to aggressive training. The techniques you will learn here are the same ones we teach law enforcement and military personnel around the world. The average training time for this level (assuming at least two training sessions per week) is nine months.

This section introduces the following material:

COMBATIVES

The combative techniques described in the Blue Belt curriculum include more-advanced techniques, especially kicks that move beyond the basics Krav Maga emphasizes. The reasons for including these "fancy" techniques are:

1. Because other systems use them, we must be proficient enough to train how to defend them.

2. Increased ability to perform these techniques tends to improve the basic techniques as well. Sweeps are a method of taking the attacker to the ground by kicking or "sweeping" his legs out from under him.

DEFENSES

This section features more defenses against kicks, and introduces defenses against three types of weapons: sticks, knives, and guns.

STICK DEFENSE

A "stick" is the most obvious member of a family of weapons known as blunt objects. These can include not only baseball bats, pool cues, tire irons, and "Club" car security devices, but also handheld rocks, hammers, and any other striking instrument that does not possess a long, sharp edge or point. Although some of these weapons (such as a rock) do not create the distance-related dangers of a stick, the defense remains the same for all of these weapons.

Of all the standard blunt objects, the stick (and its obvious synonyms, such as a baseball bat) offers the attacker one significant advantage: reach. A logical approach to stick defense must include a movement (i.e., bursting in) to eliminate this advantage. This idea of bursting forward should be strongly emphasized in any stick defense. However, you cannot assume you will always have time to burst in. Your defense must also work if you are late and must deal with the stick itself. Therefore, the following principles also apply:

1. Against an overhead attack, the defense must create no angle against the stick. This is done by keeping the elbows in tight and stabbing toward the inside of the wrist.

2. Against a baseball bat swing, the defending straight arm must be held so that the meaty part of the arm, not the elbow, is facing the stick, and the opposite hand must be up to protect the face.

It's important to know how to take away a stick, but only for tactical reasons. In other words, you might want the stick as a weapon against additional attackers. But as long as you stay close to your attacker, the stick in his hand represents little or no danger to you. Therefore, don't worry about the takeaway until you've perfected the defense.

KNIFE DEFENSES

Of the three basic weapons (gun, edged weapon, blunt object), the edged weapon or knife represents the most difficult to defend (assuming, of course, that all three are within reach). Small changes in the attack require relatively large changes in the necessary defense.

Unlike a gun, a knife cannot be grabbed. Unlike a stick, a knife still represents a significant danger even when you move in close. If you have enough distance, kicking is preferred, allowing you to keep distance from the knife. Techniques in this level will deal with kicks against the knife. The general rule for kick defenses against the knife is that when the knife is low, kick high; when the knife is high, kick low.

One prerequisite for understanding knife defenses is a basic understanding of common ways to hold the knife. The three basic holds are regular (overhead) stab, underhand stab, and straight stab (pictured below).

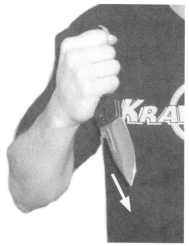
Regular (overhead) stab

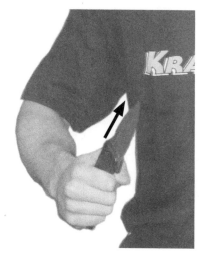
Underhand stab

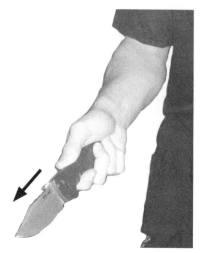
Straight stab

GUN DEFENSES

A handgun clearly represents a dangerous threat. In any situation in which you feel that compliance will result in your safety, you should comply. No possession is worth your life. However, it's possible that you may comply with every order and still get kidnapped or killed. In these circumstances, you must know an effective defense against threats with a handgun.

It's important to understand that most crimes in which a gun is involved take place within three to five feet of the defender. Gunmen come close either to terrorize, to intimidate, or to hide their actions from bystanders. This statistic indicates that the average gun-related crime offers the possibility for defensive tactics.

The over-arching principle in Krav Maga's defenses against handgun threats is this: Once you are out of the line of fire, do not go back in. Every technique prescribes to this basic principle. In addition, all Krav Maga techniques adhere to the following four stages:

1. Redirect the Line of Fire

2. Control the Weapon

3. Counterattack

4. Disarm

Often, two of these elements (usually, Control and Counterattack) overlap. As with all Krav Maga techniques, these defenses must work under stress. They must also work if simple variations are presented so that the smallest number of techniques work against the largest number of possibilities.

MENTALITY OF THE ATTACKER

Gun threats are not made in a vacuum. A gunman who sticks a gun in your face wants something. It may be your possessions, the satisfaction of humiliating you, or the thrill of terrorizing another human being. Whatever the particular motivation, the gunman who threatens you generally does so to elicit some desired response, not simply to execute you. This affords us the opportunity to make a defense. In advanced training, you may deal with situations in which the gunman may indeed be drawing a weapon simply to fire. But this belt level deals with basic gun threats in a robbery/takeover scenario.

REACTION

If you ask people what the defender is "racing" against when trying to make a defense, most people will answer, "The act of the gunman pulling the trigger." This is incorrect. The defender is not racing against the trigger pull. If that were true, every gun defense would fail.

The defender is, in fact, racing against the gunman's overall response time: the recognition that he should pull the trigger plus the trigger pull. Therefore, gun defenses, especially the initial redirections, must involve the least detectable motions possible. The techniques that follow adhere to these principles, yet offer defenses against every common type of gun threat.

CAVALIERS

"Cavaliers" are wrist locks. Why do we call them cavaliers? This was Imi's word for them. He thought they were fancy moves, and the word "cavalier" sounded fancy to him!

GROUNDFIGHTING

More-advanced techniques are covered to improve your position while on the ground.

TAKEDOWNS

Krav Maga, as a system, doesn't teach many takedowns and, admittedly, some other systems teach takedowns much more thoroughly than we do. There are any number of takedown possibilities, including single-leg, double-leg, and trip takedowns. Since Krav Maga's mandate is to keep the system simple, we present only three basic takedowns here.

Before continuing, it's important to discuss context: Why train to take someone down in the first place? One important reason is to learn to defend against takedowns. Even if you don't want to take the bad guy to the floor, he might want to take you there. In order to defend effectively, your partner has to make an adequate realistic attack.

Another reason is control. You may with to subdue someone (a drunk friend, an emotionally disturbed acquaintance) without hurting them. Taking them to the ground and holding them there is one possible way.

Finally, you may find yourself in a fight with someone who is better than you at standup fighting. If you're unable to run away, a takedown may be a way to neutralize his standup skills.

The downside to takedowns is, of course, that you will often end up on the ground yourself. Once you're on the ground, you become vulnerable to secondary attackers, and it takes just a little longer to disengage, get up, and run away.

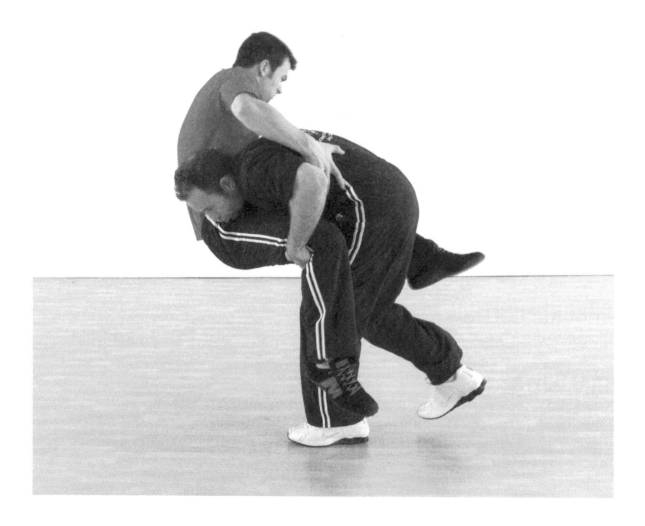

Inside and outside chops are made against narrow targets, such as the side of the neck when the chin is down and the shoulder is up. The outside chop is very similar to a hammerfist.

STARTING POSITION: Left-leg-forward fighting stance, facing a target that is in front of you.

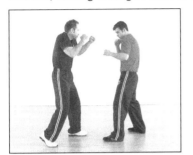

1. Raise your right hand, palm down, and extend your fingers, flexing them slightly to create tension.

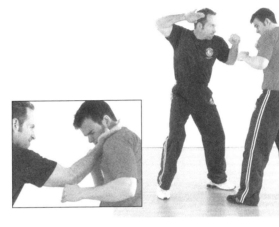

2. Moving your arm at a downward diagonal, rotate your palm sharply and strike the target with the outside (pinky) edge of your hand. Pivot your hips for power.

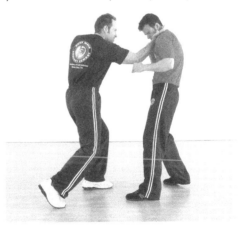

OUTSIDE CHOP

Combatives

STARTING POSITION: Left-leg-forward fighting stance, facing a target that is to your right.

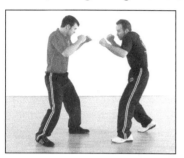

1. Raise your right hand, palm down, and extend your fingers, flexing them slightly to create tension.

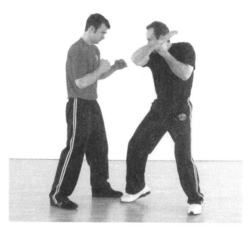

2. Strike the target with the outside (pinky) edge of your hand. Pivot your hips for power.

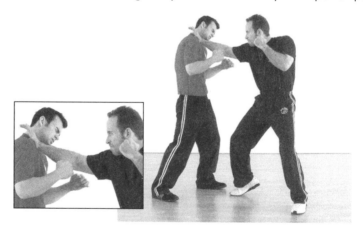

This punch is made with the top of the fist where the thumb and index finger meet. In many ways, it can be considered the opposite of a hammerfist punch. The punch is made on either an upward or lateral angle from the outside inward or forward.

STARTING POSITION: Left-leg-forward fighting stance, facing a target that is in front of you. Make a fist.

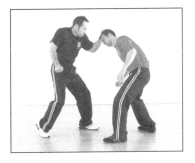

1. Swing your hand forward and upward, making sure to bring your shoulder forward and pivot your hip.

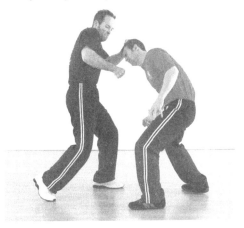

2. On contact, bend your elbow to protect it from hyperextension and to deliver extra power.

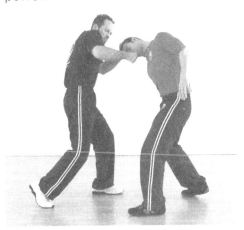

AXE KICK

Combatives

Axe kick is considered one of the less practical kicks in Krav Maga because it requires greater flexibility and exposes the kicker to danger. However, it is useful in certain situations and does have solid applications in groundfighting.

STARTING POSITION: Left-leg-forward fighting stance, facing a target.

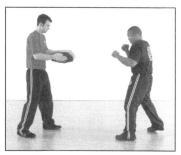

1. Raise your rear leg just across and outside the target (e.g., if you kick with your right leg, raise it toward the left).

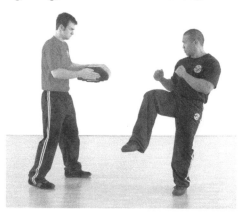

2–3. Keeping your leg relatively straight, bring it up over the target, then down hard, making contact with your heel. As you make contact, bend your knee to protect the joint and to add power. Be sure your weight is in the kick by pressing forward and down with your hip.

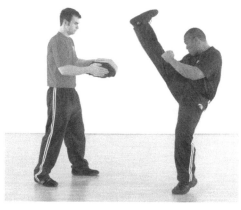

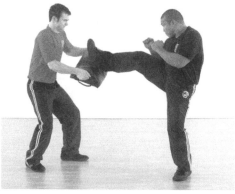

VARIATION: This version generally requires even more flexibility than the one detailed above: Rather than lifting your leg to the side, chamber your leg in tight, raise your knee high, then kick outward toward the target before delivering the axe kick downward.

This spinning kick can be used to give an opponent a "different" look if the opponent is used to dealing with round kicks and front kicks. The kick is most easily delivered if the target is slightly off-angle (e.g., if you're in a fighting stance with your right leg back and your target is to the front and left) because it requires less rotation. It is certainly possible, however, to make the kick with a full 360° spin.

STARTING POSITION: Left-leg-forward fighting stance, facing a target.

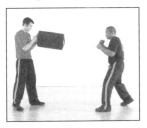

1. Pivot on your forward (left) foot so you turn over your right shoulder. Focus on bringing your head and right shoulder around so that your shoulder passes the target.

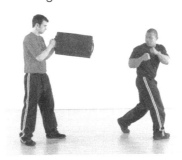

2. As your head comes around and your shoulder comes in line with the target, bring your right knee up to your chest.

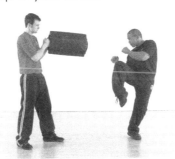

3. As your shoulder passes the target, give an Outside Slap Kick (page 167).

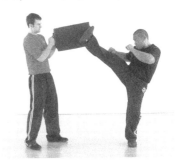

4. Land in fighting stance facing the target.

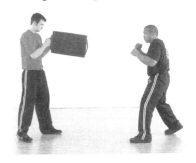

TIPS

Before turning, you can take a small diagonal step forward to decrease the degree of your turn.

SPINNING HEEL KICK

Combatives

Spinning heel kick is one of the most difficult kicks to learn. It involves a certain amount of comfort/trust in one's own body movement. However, spinning heel kick may be considered slightly more practical than spinning outside slap kick because the weapon (the heel) tends to be harder than the side of the foot, and because the kick requires slightly less spin to be delivered with strength.

STARTING POSITION: Left-leg-forward fighting stance, facing a target.

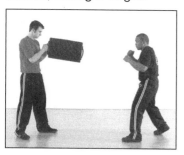

1. Take a diagonal step with your forward (left) foot. This step helps the kick by shortening the degree of the turn.

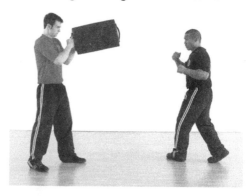

2. Spin toward your right, pivoting on your left foot. Focus on getting your head and shoulder around quickly.

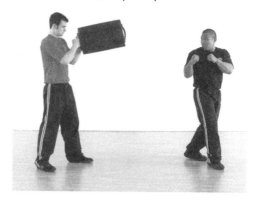

3. When your right shoulder is pointing at the target, raise your right leg and swing through to deliver a heel kick.

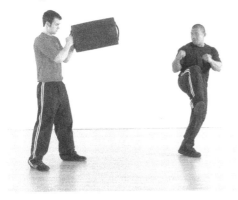

4. Strike through the target with your heel.

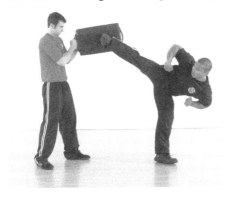

5. End in fighting stance facing the target.

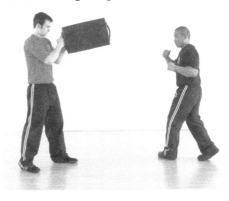

More advanced students can omit the initial diagonal step.

VARIATION: The initial diagonal step can be accompanied by a left punch to disguise it. If the instructions above are too complex, you can try this training method.

1. Make a regular Heel Kick (page 165) with your right leg.

2. Now cross your right leg over your left, then deliver the same heel kick. This "crossed" position is exactly how you should feel during a spinning heel kick just before your leg is released.

Now you can begin in a fighting stance and practice spinning (without the kick) until your shoulder points at the target (you can reach out to touch the target to confirm how far you've spun). You should end up in exactly the same position you were in when doing the "crossed" heel kick.

SWEEP WITH FORWARD KICK

Combatives

This is a "true" sweep that relies on positioning, balance, and leverage. For context, assume the following: The dynamics of the fight have taken you to a position at your opponent's side, with you either facing perpendicular to him, or almost the same direction he faces.

STARTING POSITION: Stand with the attacker on your right side, both of you facing forward.

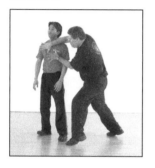

1. Control the attacker's upper body by grabbing his shirt or catching across his chest.

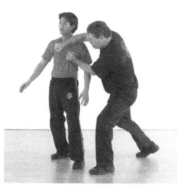

2. As you raise your right (inside) leg back, pull him so that his weight falls onto his near foot.

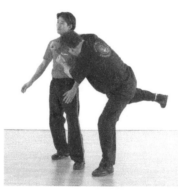

3. Sweep your right foot low so that the sole of your foot brushes the floor and the front of your ankle touches the back of his ankle. Your toes must point in the same direction as his.

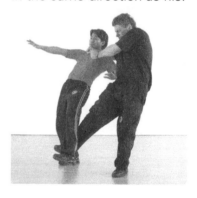

4. Continue to sweep through, letting your foot rise off the floor after contact with his ankle. At the same time, use your right arm to drive him back and down to the floor.

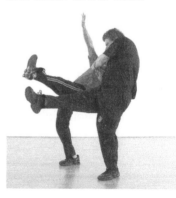

STARTING POSITION: Left-leg-forward fighting stance, facing the attacker. Grab your attacker with one hand on either of his shoulders. Your outside foot (left) must be at least on the same line as his. If you're too far away, you'll end up getting swept yourself.

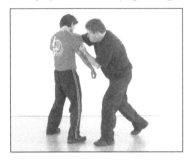

1. Using your hands on his shoulders, pull his right shoulder while pushing his left shoulder. This will force him slightly back, while also putting weight on the closest (right) leg.

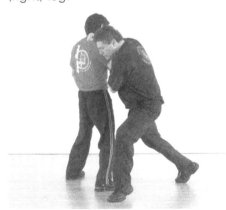

2–3. Take your right foot outside and past his right foot, and sweep backwards with a movement very similar to an offensive back kick. The sole of your foot should brush the floor; the back of your ankle should make contact with the back of his; your toes should be pointed in the opposite direction as his. Your hip should be slightly inside of his. Think about lifting your heel to the ceiling. Follow through with the motion, continuing the pull/push action with your hands and driving the attacker's upper body down.

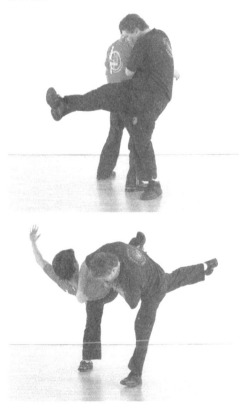

Defenses

Krav Maga has a "general" defense against medium to high attacks. This defense can be made when the hands are up or down, and especially when the defender cannot instantly determine the height of the attack. Although this defense is very basic, it is applied in defenses such as Stick (Baseball Bat Swing), Knife (Slash), Heel Kick, Spinning Heel Kick, and Round Kick, as described here.

STARTING POSITION: Left-leg-forward fighting stance.

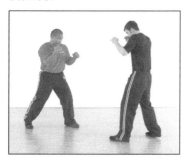

1. As the attacker throws a high right round kick, angle your body inward (if necessary) so that your shoulder points at the kick. Raising your left shoulder to protect your chin, straighten your left arm down and tighten the muscles. The back of your hand should face the kick so that your elbow is not exposed. Simultaneously bring your right hand up and across to protect your face. Be sure your chin is tucked.

Continue with counters such as an elbow to the face.

TIPS

If time allows, burst in to meet the kick before it develops full power. Even if time does not allow for a step, you should still lean in to brace yourself against the kick.

The defense can be made with the straight arm in either a fist or with fingers extended. A fist is preferable because it tightens up the arm muscles to help them absorb the impact. However, if you are surprised, the "fingers extended" version is probably what you'll do.

Once you've blocked, it is also possible to trap the leg and deliver knees, or sweep.

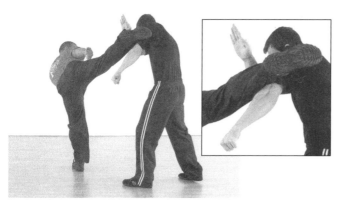

Defenses

In addition to stopping high kicks, as shown in the General Defense against Medium to High Kicks (page 230), Krav Maga also utilizes a redirecting (in this case, "sliding") defense against high round kicks.

STARTING POSITION: Left-leg-forward fighting stance with your hands a bit low to simulate either setting up the opponent or fatigue.

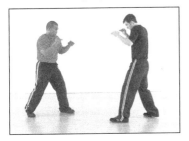

1. As the attacker throws a high right round kick, stab just beneath the rising kick with your left hand, which is in a fist with the palm facing the floor. At the same time, bring your other hand up and across to protect your face.

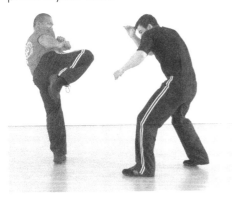

2–3. Quickly raise your arm as you feel the kick slide along your arm, and simultaneously burst forward diagonally in the direction of the kick. The attacker's leg should be driven up, decreasing its power and stretching out the attacker's groin.

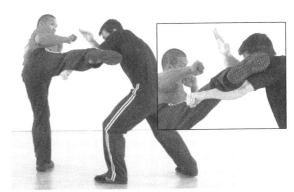

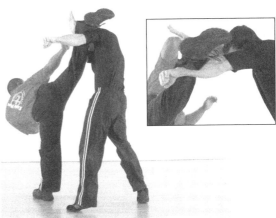

From here, you can a) throw the attacker off, b) trap the leg and punch, or c) trap the leg and perform an Outside Sweep with Heel Kick.

TIPS

The same defense can be made if the hands are down.

Be aware that if the technique is performed late, the "slide" will not be achieved, and the movement becomes a General Defense.

Defenses

This defense can be made to the live or dead side, using either hand. However, it is generally easier to make to the attacker's live side because it allows the defender to pluck at the attacker's foot, rather than at the heel. It is also easier to defend on the defender's live side because it makes the body defense simpler (the hips are already turned). However, these two angles are not always offered at the same time.

STARTING POSITION: Left-leg-forward fighting stance.

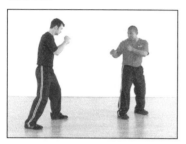

1. As the attacker throws a medium right side kick, reach out with your right hand, making sure your hand and forearm travel parallel to the floor so that they do not offer an angle to the kick.

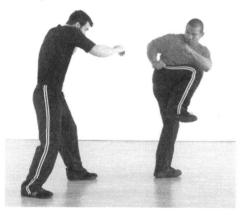

2–3. As your hand passes the approaching kick, pluck backwards, letting your elbow and forearm slide tight along your body. Allow the motion of the pluck to pull your body forward (with the left side leading), making a

body defense. Simultaneously burst in with your feet.

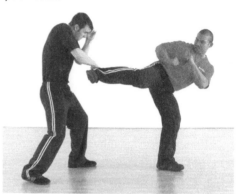

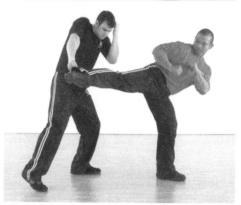

Continue with counterattacks.

TIPS

This technique must be made quickly— the defending hand moves in a quick "pickpocket" motion. If you defend to your dead side, you will need to take a step with your back foot in order to burst in.

The principles and dynamics of this defense are exactly the same as those in Sliding Defense against High Round Kick (page 231).

STARTING POSITION: Left-leg-forward fighting stance.

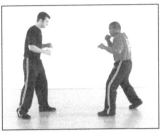

1. As the attacker makes a right spinning heel kick, burst diagonally forward, bringing your left hand across your face and forward to protect against the kick (if you're late) or against a spinning backfist or elbow. Your advance should take you toward the attacker's right hip as it comes around in the spin.

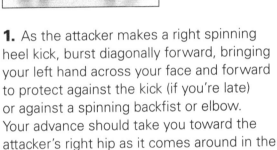

2. Stab with your right arm, aiming to slide just underneath the knee.

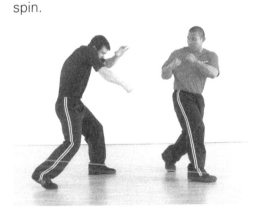

3. As your arm makes contact, raise it up to take the momentum from the kick.

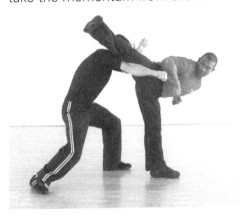

If you succeed in catching the leg, you can a) trap it and strike, b) throw the person off by shoving the leg into the air, or c) trap the leg and perform a sweep.

Defenses

Although a fighting stance is used to describe the kick in this lesson, this defense can be performed from a fighting stance or a neutral stance. This defense assumes that you identify the attack relatively early.

STARTING POSITION: Left-leg-forward fighting stance.

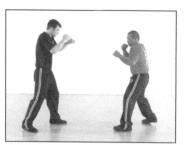

1–2. As the attacker makes a right spinning heel kick, make a defensive front kick with your right leg. Kick the attacker on the leg just below the right buttock, at the top of his thigh. Be sure your hands are up and covering in case the kick comes high and your defense is too late to catch the attacker's leg.

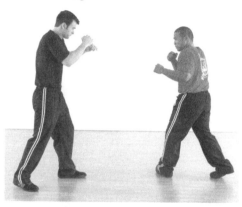

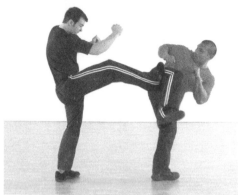

"Overhead swing" refers to almost any attack in which the swing is coming from a point higher than the attacker's shoulder in a downward motion. The attack might be straight down or at a slight angle.

Note: *Whenever in doubt, use this defense as your "default" defense. It offers the most overall protection.*

STARTING POSITION: Neutral or passive stance.

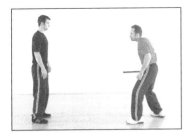

1. As the attacker swings the stick using his right arm, bring your hands up to your head, keeping your fingers extended and the blades of your hands downward. Be sure your elbows are in tight to your body so that your defending arm is straight and presents no angle to the stick. Bring your head down but keep your eyes forward. Lean forward with your body even before your feet move. This small motion will help get you past the stick.

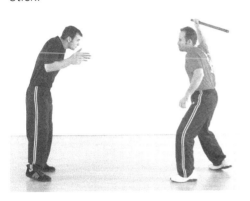

2. Stab out with your defending (usually the left) hand to the inside of the attacker's wrist and burst forward with your feet. At the same time, punch to the attacker's face with your other hand. As you stab and punch, keep your shoulders square to the attacker. This keeps your head from being exposed.

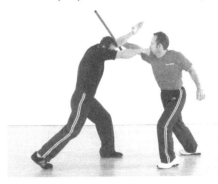

3. As soon as you feel the defense has been made, immediately grab the attacker's shoulder with both hands and deliver knee strikes.

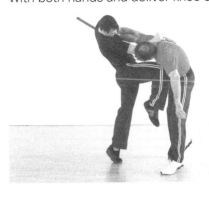

continued on next page

continued from previous page

TIPS

If you are late stabbing out your defending hand, you will defend the stick instead. As long as you haven't created an angle against the stick, you should be all right.

VARIATIONS: Once you understand the basic defense, have the attacker swing at different angles. Be sure you always stab just inside the swinging hand and not automatically straight overhead.

TAKEAWAY 1: If you feel the assailant weaken, slide your left hand along his right arm until it reaches the hand. If you feel the tip of the stick protrude from his hand, clasp it and pull while giving a palm heel strike to the side of his head with your right hand.

TAKEAWAY 2 (NOT PICTURED): Reach back with your left hand, grab the end of the stick, and make a sharp "U" shape with it to pop the other end out of the attacker's hand.

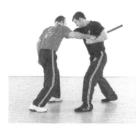 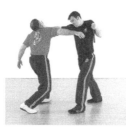

In almost every case, it is preferable to defend overhead swings on the live side. However, if the attack comes at an extreme angle (for instance, if a right-handed attacker swings from the defender's far right side), the defender may have no choice but to make an off-angle, or dead-side, defense.

STARTING POSITION: Neutral or passive stance.

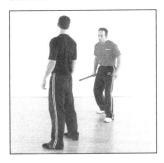

1–2. As the attacker swings the stick toward your right using his right arm, raise your near-side (right) hand and stab to the outside of the attacker's wrist, making sure not to create an angle against the stick. As you raise your hand, turn your shoulders to square them to the attacker and lean forward to get in past the stick. Step with your outside (left) foot to burst forward and close more distance.

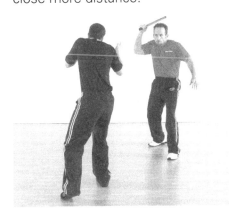

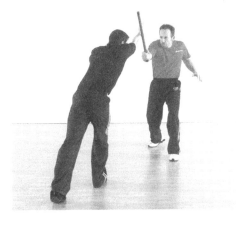

3. As you redirect the stick, pivot in the direction of the stick, trapping or covering the stick.

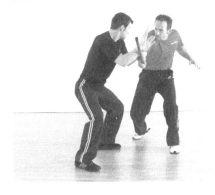

steps 4–7 continued on next page

Stick Defenses

continued from previous page

4–7. Catch the arm and counterattack with punches; disarm the attacker.

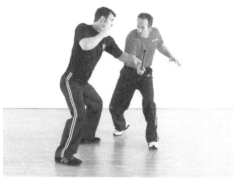

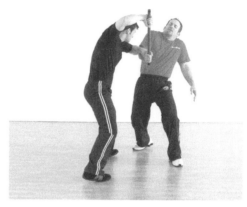

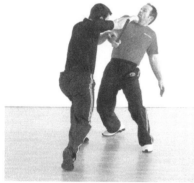

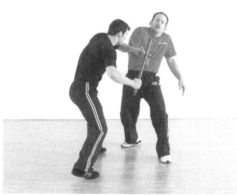

VARIATION: Burst in with your inside (right) foot instead of your left. As you redirect the stick, take a step with your left foot and counterattack. This defense puts more distance between the defender and a possible third party approaching from behind.

Unlike overhead swing, in which the defense redirects the attack, this defense stops the attack. However, we still emphasize leaning forward and bursting in. Also, note again that if you are ever in doubt as to whether the attack is an overhead or baseball bat swing, use the Stick Defense against Overhead Swing (page 235).

STARTING POSITION: Neutral or passive stance.

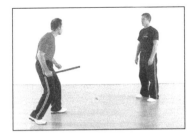

1. As the attacker swings the stick toward your left using his right arm, turn your left shoulder in and toward the direction of the stick. As you do this, lean in toward the attacker's arm/shoulder and extend your left arm down along your body, but not touching. Be sure the meaty part of your arm, not the elbow, is pointed toward the oncoming stick. Also bring your right hand across your body and up to protect the left side of your face. Note that this is very much like the General Defense against Medium to High Kicks (page 230).

2. Burst forward toward the inside of the stick. On impact, "pop" your left arm slightly forward for additional impact against the body or, if you are defending against the stick itself, to catch the stick earlier in its motion.

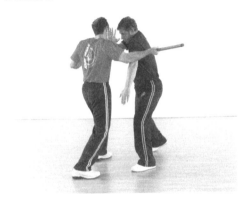

steps 3–4 continued on next page

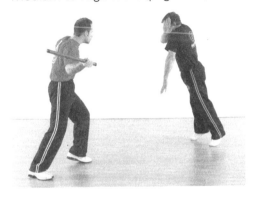

continued from previous page

3. After impact, immediately bring your left hand up to trap the stick arm while simultaneously giving a right elbow strike to the attacker's face.

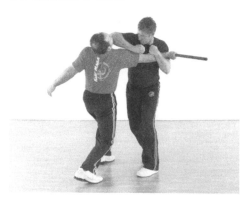

4. Follow up with knee strikes.

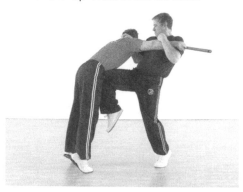

TIPS

Even though your left arm is extended downward, be sure your left shoulder is up to help protect your jaw.

Sometimes you will not have time to burst forward. This is why turning inward is so important—it often takes you forward, past the stick, even if your feet don't move.

TAKEAWAY VARIATION: Once you feel the attacker weaken, reach over with your right hand, grab the end of the stick, and snap it downward in a "U."

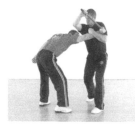
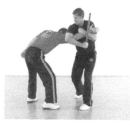
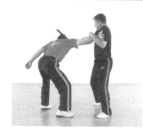

Like all kick defenses, this defense assumes the attacker is at a distance and is approaching with determination. If you don't recognize the attack early on, you won't be able to kick.

In previous years, we made a distinction among different attacks and executed different types of kicks relative to each grip. However, emphasis was always placed on delivering ANY kind of kick as early as possible. More recently, we've simplified the technique to follow that strategy so that you deliver one midline kick against all attacks. This obeys the dictum that you will probably not see a knife anyway, and therefore you won't be able to judge the type of hold. There is no time for decision making—just send a kick!

STARTING POSITION: Neutral or passive stance.

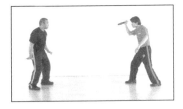

1–2. As the attacker approaches, burst forward with a kick similar to a Defensive Front Kick (page 97), or Front Kick—Vertical Target (page 46).

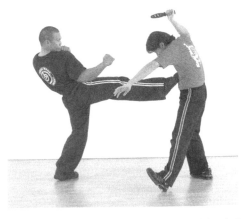

Immediately make distance and look for an object to use as a weapon or shield, or run.

TIPS

If there is no time to advance, make the kick in place. In either case, make yourself as long as possible by extending your hip. This allows you to strike while the knife is as far away as possible.

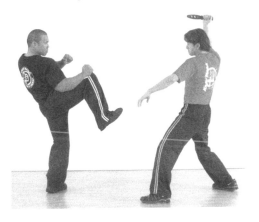

VARIATION: Continue to attack in order to destroy the target, controlling the knife arm with your hands.

KICK AGAINST STRAIGHT STAB (BAILING OUT)

Kick Defenses

This defense can be used if the defender recognizes the knife attack and wants to bail out and away from the line of the attack. If the defender does not recognize in advance that a straight-stab knife attack is coming, he should make a regular front kick as in the previous exercise.

STARTING POSITION: Neutral or passive stance.

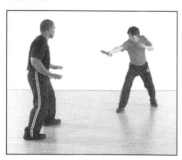

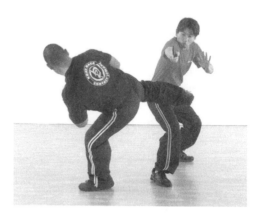

1–2. As the attacker bursts in with the stab, step diagonally forward with your left foot and "bail out" with your body, taking your right shoulder toward your left knee to get out of the line of the attacker. As you make this body defense, deliver a round kick with the ball of your foot to the attacker's groin. Recoil your foot quickly and move off, looking to escape or pick up an object to use as a shield or weapon.

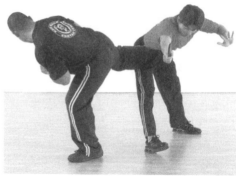

VARIATION: It is possible to continue with attacks and attempt to control the weapon. This is, however, difficult to perform in realistic scenarios, and we no longer require it as a part of the technique. However, we describe it here for reference:

After delivering the round kick, recoil your foot and chamber for a side kick. Deliver a side kick to the side of the attacker's knee while controlling the knife hand with your right hand.

Caution: In training, DO NOT let your partner put his finger on the trigger as it may get broken.

STARTING POSITION: Neutral or passive stance.

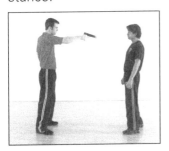

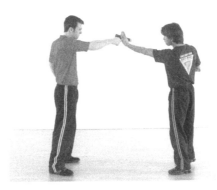

1. As the attacker presents the gun with his right hand, smoothly send your left hand to the weapon in a straight line, putting the side of your index finger at the side of the weapon and pushing in a straight line to your right. The movement should take the gun off your body parallel to the floor. Any diagonal movement up or down means that the gun stays on your body for a longer period of time. This movement also moves the weapon from vital areas (center of the chest) to areas that are less vital, until the gun is completely off. Just as your hand reaches the weapon and begins to redirect, make a body defense by allowing your left shoulder to come forward. This has the added benefit of putting your motion and weight toward the gunman even though your feet have not yet moved.

2. Grab the weapon sharply and "punch" it down so that the gun points 90° away from you and is roughly parallel with the floor. You should already be putting weight down on the weapon. Burst forward with your feet so that you end up in a fighting stance with your left foot just outside the gunman's right foot. Often, the gun will end up on the attacker's stomach. This is fine, but is not a requirement since the gunman's body position is not always predictable. A more consistent rule is this: The gun should be in front of your right thigh (but not pointing that way), with your weight on it.

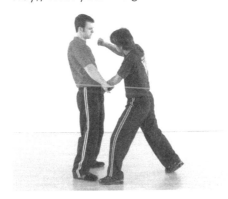

steps 3–6 continued on next page

Gun Defenses

continued from previous page

3. Keep your weight on the weapon but deliver a punch to the face with your right hand. Always make sure your weight stays on the weapon!

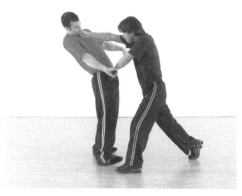

4. Recoil your punch, slide your hand along your body to avoid the line of fire, reach down, and grab the weapon at the hammer or the back of the slide.

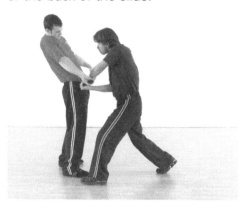

5. Rotate the gun sharply 90° to "break" it from the gunman's grasp. This may break the gunman's finger.

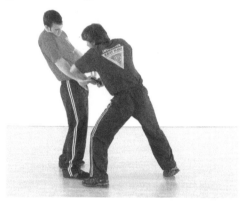

6. Pull the weapon back toward your left side. Note that your feet have not yet moved. As soon as the weapon is in your possession, retreat to a safe distance.

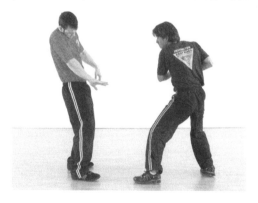

The initial redirection must involve no other body movement: no leaning, no tensing, no shifting of your feet.

As you redirect in Step 2, your right hand can already be coming up to punch, but it should be close to your body so that it is not in the line of fire.

TO THE HEAD VARIATION: This technique is the same as the regular defense against Gun from the Front (page 243), with one difference: You make an earlier body defense by moving your head even before your hand has reached the gun (although the hand always leads the motion). This is possible because the movement to get your head out of the line of fire is shorter and simpler than moving your whole body.

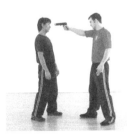
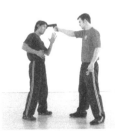
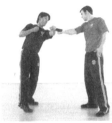

GUN TO THE SIDE OF THE HEAD

Gun Defenses

For demonstration purposes, these instructions assume that the gun is in the attacker's right hand. Except for the initial redirection, this technique is essentially like Gun from the Front (page 243).

STARTING POSITION: Neutral or passive stance, with the gunman on your left side.

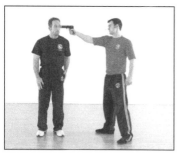

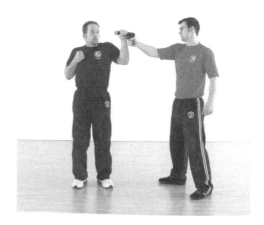

1–2. As the attacker presents the gun with his right hand, lift your left hand up along your body, keeping your elbow back. As your hand nears the gun, begin to make a body defense by tilting your head backward. The timing of this head movement is early, similar to that of Gun from the Front (To the Head). With your fingers up, redirect the gun forward and grab it.

3. Immediately turn the gun sharply so that it points approximately 90° away from you and "punch" the weapon down with your weight on top of it.

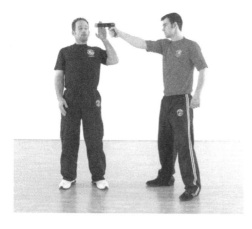

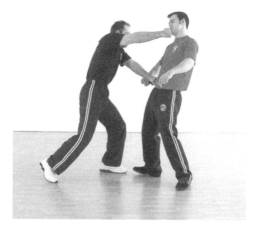

4–6. Turn your body and burst toward the attacker, completing the technique exactly as in Gun from the Front.

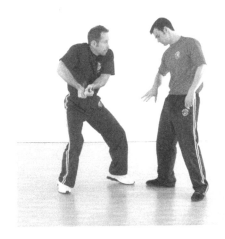

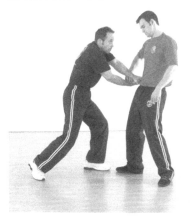

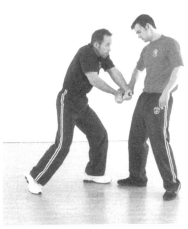

Gun Defenses

STARTING POSITION: Neutral or passive stance, with the attacker to your left.

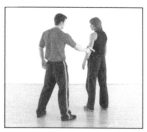

1. As the attacker puts the gun behind your left arm with his right hand, make a small redirection with your arm, pushing the gun off line behind you. This movement should be relatively small.

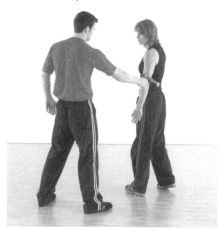

2. Turn toward the gunman and reach toward him with your left hand (the one that made the redirection), slipping your arm underneath the gunman's. Your goal should be to reach as deep as possible even before you've moved your feet.

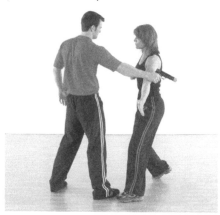

3. Continuing to reach with your left hand, burst in VERY DEEP so that your left foot is outside the gunman's right foot. Wrap your left arm up, bringing your fist tightly to your chest to secure the forearm holding the gun. With your rear arm, deliver an elbow strike to the gunman's face. As you deliver the strike, you can slide your other arm back to secure the wrist rather than the forearm.

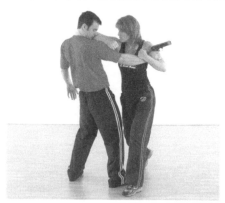

4. Follow with knee strikes.

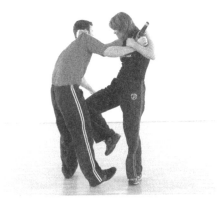

5. With your free hand, reach over, pinky up, and grab the barrel.

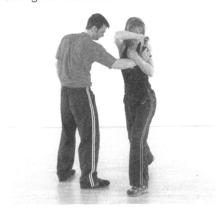

6. Snap down hard with your elbow to break his grip.

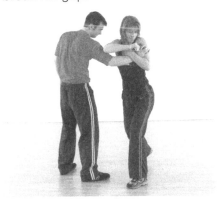

7. Lift the gun up to get it off the finger in the trigger.

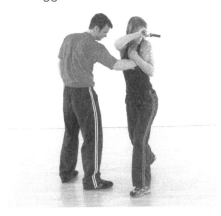

8. Strike with an elbow or the muzzle and get out, creating distance.

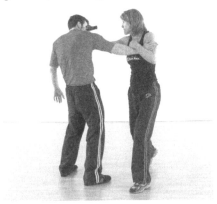

TIPS

Be sure your hold on the wrist is strong. Press your fist to your chest. Push your shoulder forward—note that this is your shoulder, not your whole upper body.

Gun Defenses

This technique is the only one in the Krav Maga system wherein you redirect, control, and disarm first, THEN counterattack. This is never the desired order of events, but there is no better movement from this position.

STARTING POSITION: Neutral or passive stance, with the attacker to your left.

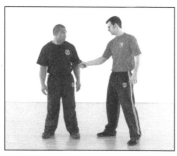

1. As the attacker puts the gun to your side (in front of your arm) with his right hand, slide your left hand up along your body with your fingers down and palm facing forward.

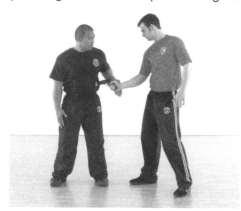

2–3. Catch the attacker's wrist (here your hand acts as a brace, preventing the wrist from bending) and push forward to redirect the weapon. At the same time, contract your abs and make a diagonal step toward the gunman.

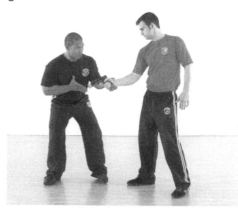

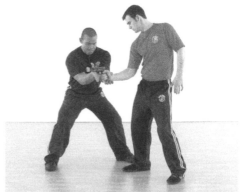

4. As you advance, slide your right hand in along your body, avoiding the line of fire, then reach forward and grab the barrel. Your fingers should be down and your thumb should be up to help prevent the gun from being turned back toward you before you have control. As you grab the gunman's wrist/hand with your left hand and the barrel with your right hand, your knees should be slightly bent to maintain balance, and you should be on the balls of your feet.

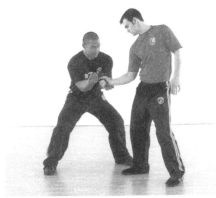

5. Pull against the wrist with your inside hand and turn your outside shoulder sharply in, rotating the gun in and slightly down. This should break the weapon from the gunman's grasp. Taking the gun slightly down presses it over the thumb, which causes additional pain.

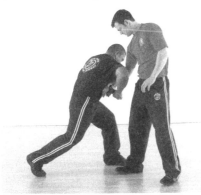

6–7. Using your right hand, pull the gun away from the gunman and toward your body. Deliver a punch to the gunman's face with your left hand, and follow with a right punch, striking with the muzzle of the gun.

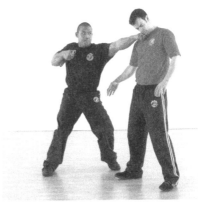

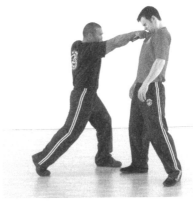

Retreat quickly to a safe distance.

GUN FROM THE FRONT, PUSHING INTO THE STOMACH

Gun Defenses

Although the basic threat here is Gun from the Front, the gunman creates difficulty if he presses the gun hard into the stomach, perhaps to push the defender backward. If the gun is pressed deeply, it will be difficult to make the regular Gun from the Front technique (page 243). In this case, apply the defense for Gun from the Side, in Front of the Arm. You will need to add a pivot of your hips to allow the gun room to move. This example assumes you shift back on your right side.

STARTING POSITION: Passive or neutral stance, with the gunman holding the gun to your stomach and pushing

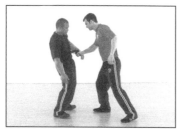

1. As the gunman pushes into your body, pivot your right hip back while your left hand slides in and redirects the gun by catching the gunman's wrist exactly as in Gun from the Side, in Front of the Arm (page 250). The gunman's push, combined with the pivot of your hip, may cause your right foot to step back. This is fine—just be sure the body motion precedes the foot step to avoid telegraphing.

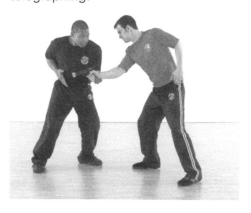

2. Slide your right hand along your body and then forward to catch the muzzle of the weapon. Be sure your elbows are tight against your body to create a strong frame and support for your grip.

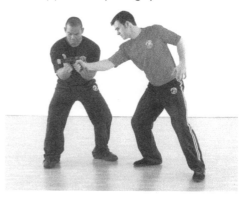

3. Disarm exactly as described in Gun from the Side, in Front of the Arm (page 250) and then continue with counterattacks.

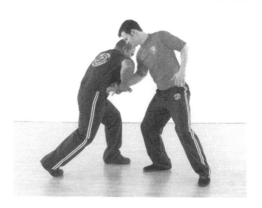

The technique for Gun from Behind is exactly the same as Gun from the Side, Behind the Arm (page 248), with a couple of small differences.

STARTING POSITION: Neutral or passive stance, with the attacker behind you.

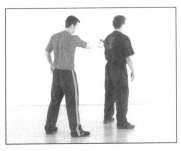

1. As the attacker puts the gun against your back with his right hand, look behind you! You aren't really concerned about what is touching your body. You need to make sure the gun isn't in the other hand.

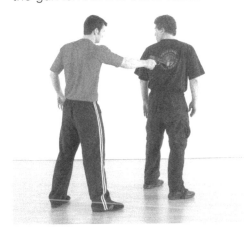

2. Leading with your left arm, turn deeply enough to redirect the weapon and take your body out of the line of fire. The body defense should cause you to immediately lean back toward the attacker even before your feet move.

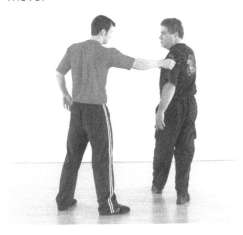

steps 3–10 continued on next page

continued from previous page

3–5. Continuing to reach with your left hand, burst in VERY DEEP so that your left foot is outside the gunman's right foot. Wrap your left arm up, bringing your fist tightly to your chest to secure the forearm holding the gun. With your rear arm, deliver an elbow strike to the gunman's face. As you deliver the strike, you can slide your other arm back to secure the wrist rather than the forearm.

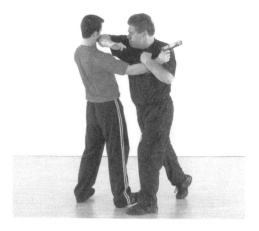

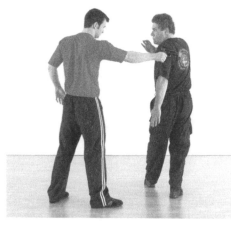

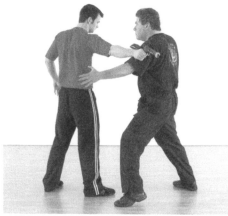

6. Follow with kicks to the groin.

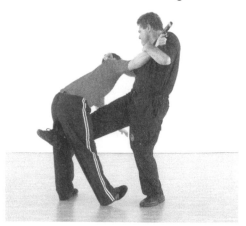

7. With your free hand, reach over, pinky up, and grab the barrel.

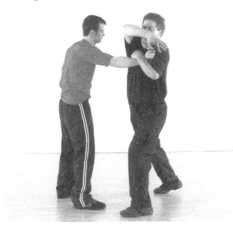

8. Snap down hard with your elbow to break his grip.

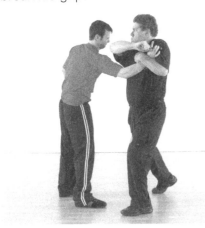

9. Lift the gun up to get it off the finger in the trigger.

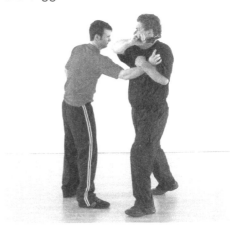

10. Strike with an elbow or the muzzle and get out, creating distance.

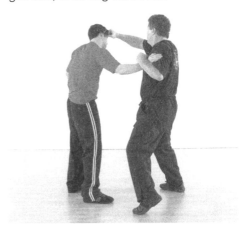

TIPS

If the gun is held low, your arm will make the redirection along with the body defense. If the gun is held high on your back, your arm will have little or no effect, and you'll mostly make a body defense. However, your arm still helps your body rotate.

Cavaliers

STARTING POSITION: Grab the attacker's right wrist with your left hand. With your right hand, "cap" the attacker's right hand by placing your hand over his. This can be done with an explosive punching movement with your hand.

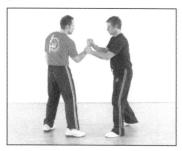

1. Pull the wrist toward you with your left and push down with your right, putting strain on the attacker's wrist. Apply pressure using your upper body and even your legs, not just your arms. This hold should take place approximately a forearm's length away from your body.

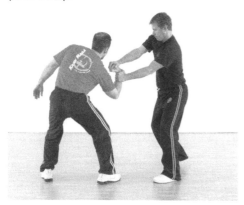

2. Pivot to your left on your right foot while driving the attacker's arm down, slamming him to the ground. As you complete the move, bend your knees, NOT your back, to keep control of the attacker.

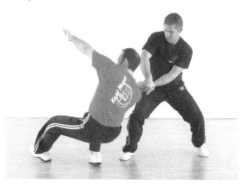

3. Immediately twist sharply back, laying your shin against his neck and your knee along his arm to prevent him from rolling out.

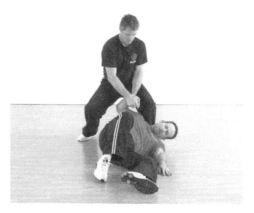

TIPS
The cavalier is made by pushing the fist down toward the wrist, not by twisting it.

STARTING POSITION: Grab the attacker's right wrist with your left hand. With your right, "cap" the attacker's right hand by placing your hand over his. This can be done with an explosive punching movement with your hand.

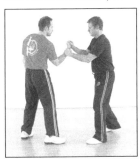

1. Pull the wrist toward you with your left and push down with your right, putting strain on the attacker's wrist. Apply the pressure using your upper body and even your legs, not just your arms. This hold should take place approximately a forearm's length away from your body for maximum force.

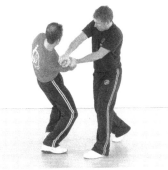

2–3. Burst forward, pushing the arm to the outside of the attacker's shoulder and then down. Be prepared to move farther forward with your feet if the attacker's fall requires it.

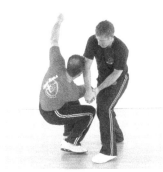

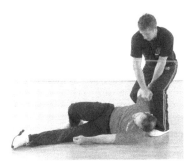

4. Immediately twist sharply back, laying your shin against his neck and your knee along his arm to prevent him from rolling out.

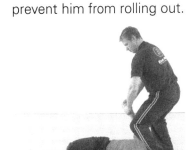

Cavaliers

This cavalier often causes the attacker's hand to open, and is effective if you wish to make him let go of an object.

This cavalier can be the same as either #1 or #2, except that instead of placing one hand on the wrist and one on the hand, both hands are on the wrist and both thumbs push the back of the hand down to make the technique.

STARTING POSITION: Catch the attacker's hand and wrist in your two hands. Place both thumbs on the back of his hand; be sure your fingers around his wrist do not brace the wrist and prevent it from bending.

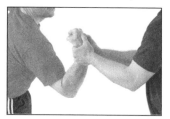

1. Pull with your fingers and push with your thumbs so the attacker's hand goes down toward his wrist. This will cause his hand to open.

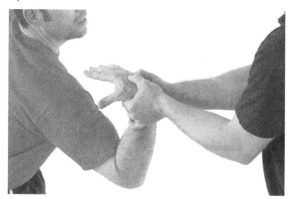

From here, you can take him down as in #1 and #2.

Cavalier #4 is made when the attacker's wrist is too strong, or when the defender wants the cavalier to knock an object out of the attacker's hand.

STARTING POSITION: Grab the attacker's right wrist with your left hand.

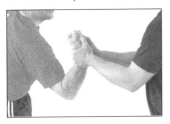

1. With your right arm, deliver an elbow strike to the attacker's wrist.

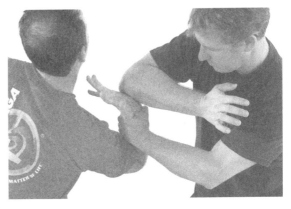

As soon as you feel that you've broken the wrist, press down with your forearm until you take the attacker down.

Groundfighting

STARTING POSITION: On your back, with the attacker straddling you and pinning your wrists to the floor with his weight.

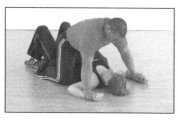

1. Buck your hips up toward your head and over to one side. At the same time, slide your hands down in an arc toward your own hips, similar to the way a child makes "snow angels." Be sure your hands slide on the ground. They should not lift up.

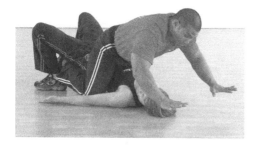

2–3. As the attacker topples off, roll over and counterattack.

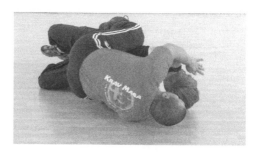

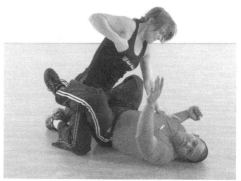

VARIATION: Before you buck, for added leverage, you can trap one of the defender's legs with your leg.

With your wrists pinned close together or crossed over your head, the "snow angel" technique does not work because you have no leverage to move your arms.

STARTING POSITION: On your back, with the attacker straddling you and pinning your wrists together to the floor, above your head, with his weight.

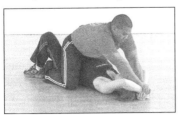

1. Move one hand so that you can trap the attacker's wrist; it does not matter which of his hands you trap. If the attacker is so strong that you cannot move one hand, you can "fake" with that hand— when he pushes down on that side, move your other hand.

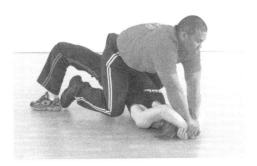

2–3. Once you trap his hand, buck your hips and execute a trap-and-roll movement to that side.

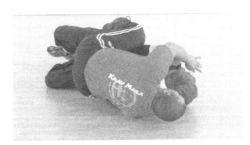

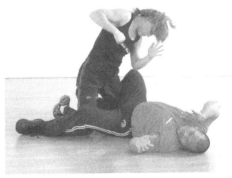

You can sometimes use your forearm/elbow against his arm for additional leverage as you buck your hips.

TIPS

Even if you cannot move your hands, you can still execute the trap and roll. Remember, by pinning your hands close over your head, he has also trapped his own hand in a position that makes it difficult for him to base out. The trap and roll will work! However, he may release his grip and base out, which means your wrists are free and you can work on a standard trap-and-roll.

CHOKE WHILE ATTACKER IS IN GUARD

Groundfighting

Some attackers, when punching from the guard, will overcommit their weight to the punch. While this is an effective technique, it encourages the defender to grapple rather than get up.

STARTING POSITION: On your back, the attacker in your guard.

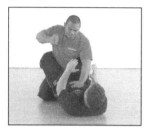

1–2. As the attacker makes a right punch, redirect it so that it passes by your head to your opposite (right) shoulder. Use his momentum, plus the strength of your legs pulling in, to bring him in close.

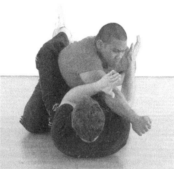

3. Wrap your outside hand around his neck and grab the biceps of your redirecting arm. Bend the redirecting arm back and grab your own head.

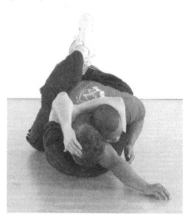

4. Squeeze.

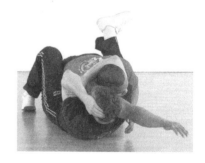

VARIATION: You can also use your head for additional pressure by pushing in.

This movement is a variation of the Arm Bar (page 196) discussed in Green Belt. It is made when you have the opponent in your guard. It is especially effective if the attacker tries to escape the guard by sliding one arm between his body and your leg.

STARTING POSITION: On your back, the attacker in your guard.

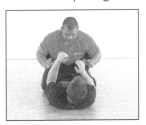

1–2. When the opponent tries to escape the guard by slipping his left arm under your right leg, grab hold of his other arm above the elbow. At the same time, shift your hips so your body pivots toward your right. Your goal is to be perpendicular to your opponent. Bring your right leg across the back of his neck. Keep a tight hold on the left arm.

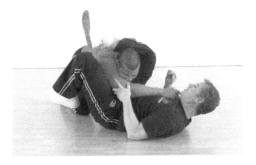

3. Bring the left leg up and cross it over the top of the right foot. The right foot must reach the crook of the top leg. Squeeze.

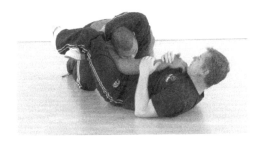

If the attacker resists, or your hold isn't strong enough, reach up with a free hand and grab the back of his head, bending it inward.

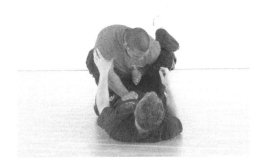

VARIATION: If the hold does not seem to be working, you can always punch to his face.

Groundfighting

You can make this attack on its own, but it also works well if you try the "Sit Up and Sweep" technique (page 198) and then transition to this attack if that one fails.

STARTING POSITION: On your back, attacker in your closed guard.

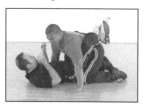

1. When the attacker sits back in your guard, sit up and uncross your ankles; put your left hand on the ground and reach your right hand up and across as though trying to reach past his right shoulder.

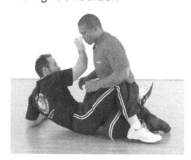

2. Wrap your right arm around the back of his neck and then under his chin.

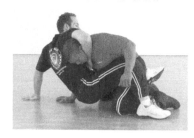

3. Grab your right hand with your left (you may need to scoot your hips back a little to do this).

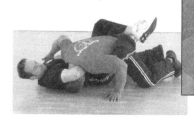

4. Wrap your legs around his waist again, crossing your ankles, and lie back.

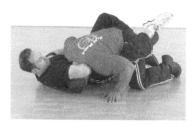

5. Pull with your arms, sealing the choke, and push away with your legs to stretch him out.

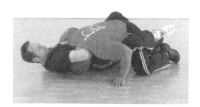

If you find yourself in someone else's guard, they may attempt a guillotine against you. Here are two basic defenses against a guillotine. First, avoid the guard. If you feel the attacker attempt the guillotine, hop out of his guard, moving to the same side as the attacking arm. If you cannot escape the guard, make the following defense:

STARTING POSITION: Attacker holds you in his guard while he snakes his right arm around your neck.

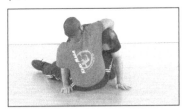

1. The minute you feel the attacker wrap his arm around your neck, tuck your chin. With your left hand, pluck at his hands to relieve some pressure. At the same time, wrap your right arm around his neck. This makes it difficult for him to stretch you out with his legs.

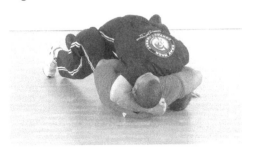

2. Lift your hips up and spread your feet wide to "stack up"; think about creating a tripod with your two feet, using your right arm and shoulder as the third foot of the tripod.

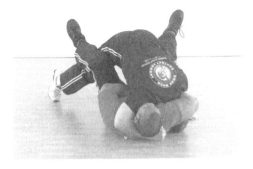

3. Using your body weight, drive your shoulder into the attacker's neck and throat. It will be very difficult for him to maintain the guillotine.

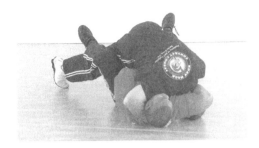

steps 4–7 continued on next page

Groundfighting

continued from previous page

4–7. When he releases his arms, either sit back on your knees (still in his guard) or hop out of his guard to side mount if possible (shown).

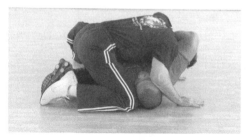

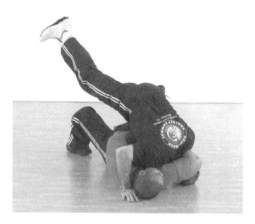

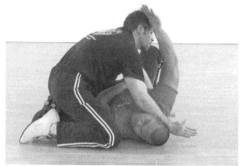

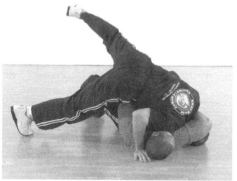

While Krav Maga does not emphasize many grappling or submission moves, the rear headlock (also called a "carotid choke" or "rear naked choke") is good to know. You may need to use it, and it is always good to attack properly when your partner is learning to defend. The basic points here apply whether you are on top or bottom from behind.

STARTING POSITION: On your back, with the attacker on top of you but with his back to you.

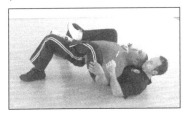

1. Wrap your legs around his body and dig your heels into his thighs just below the groin. This is known as getting your "hooks" in; the position makes it difficult for the attacker to perform an escape. Wrap your right arm around his neck so that his throat is in the crook of your elbow.

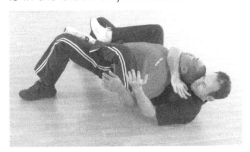

2. Grab your left bicep with your right hand.

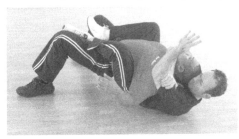

3. Put your left hand on the left side of your head. Squeeze your elbows together and puff out your chest. The idea is to simultaneously squeeze your forearm on one side of his neck and your bicep on the other side of his neck, applying pressure to the carotid arteries in his neck and temporarily cutting off the blood supply to his brain.

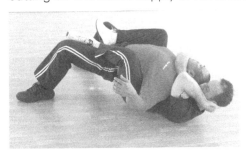

Groundfighting

This position refers to a hold in which the attacker is on his back placing a bar arm or carotid hold on the defender. The attacker will also generally have his heels hooked into the defender's legs. Note how principles and movements from the standing headlock apply on the ground as well.

STARTING POSITION:
Attacker is on his back, with defender face up in attacker's guard.

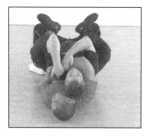

1. As the attacker begins the headlock, turn your chin away from the attacking side to relieve the pressure of the choke. Send both hands up and backward to pluck at the attacker's joined hands.

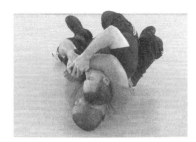

2. With your feet, drive your shoulders up and back toward the attacker's shoulder on the holding side (i.e., if his right arm is around your throat, drive up toward his right shoulder). Continue driving until your head and/or shoulders touch the floor on that side. Shift your hips to the side. Your goal is to get your hips and rear flat to the floor—even if this means lying on top of his leg. At this point, the headlock is gone.

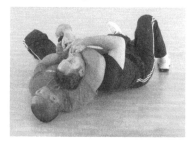

3–4. Turn sharply inward; you will most likely end up on top in the attacker's guard or side mount. Follow up with counterattacks.

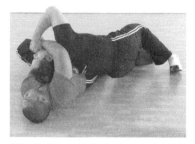

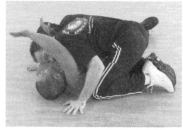

Because of the ground position, reaching your hands up and back will probably have less effect on the attacker than the standing version. Your goal is relieve some pressure.

This is a simple takedown that relies very little on technique.

STARTING POSITION: Left-leg-forward fighting stance, facing the attacker.

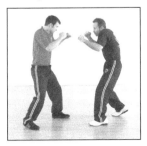

1. Get in close, drop low, and wrap your arms around your opponent's legs, with your head and/or shoulder in his stomach. Your arms may be clasped, or you can hook one hand around each of his legs.

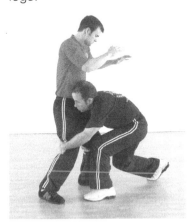

2–3. Pull his legs in toward you and left slightly; at the same time, use your legs to drive your weight into his stomach.

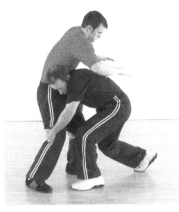

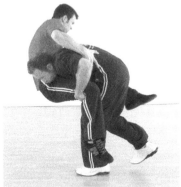

4. If you wish to continue the attack on the ground, immediately move upward onto his body and continue to attack; you may also try to disengage and stand up while he is still on the ground.

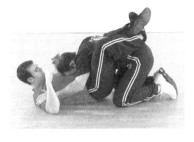

TIPS

This simple takedown is more easily defended by the opponent. He can sprawl or simply push down on your head to stop your forward progress. However, it's a good, generally effective takedown against a non-expert opponent.

TAKEDOWN #2: DOUBLE-LEG TAKEDOWN

Takedowns

This takedown is still simple but requires a little more technique. In this example, we are moving slightly to the attacker's right side.

STARTING POSITION: Left-leg-forward fighting stance, facing the attacker.

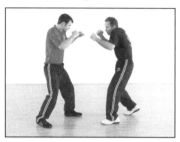

1. Drop low and shoot in quickly, wrapping your arms around your opponent's legs; you must get your hips in close with your feet underneath you. Keep your hands up as you approach to guard against a knee to the face. Your head may be to the outside of his right hip (see note below).

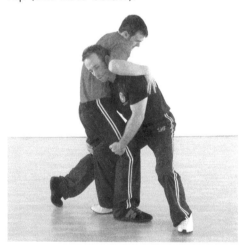

2. With your hips underneath you, use your legs to lift the attacker slightly off the ground (he doesn't have to go high; just get his feet off the floor). Use your arms to sweep his legs to your left; at the same time, use your head to push or steer his upper body to your right.

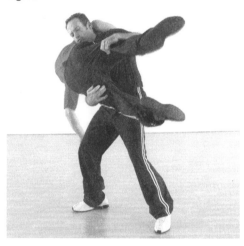

3. As the attacker goes to the floor, you should find yourself in a side mount position.

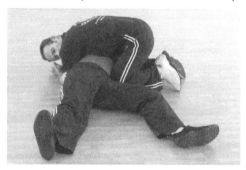

TIPS

It is very important to get your hips close to the attacker and under your shoulders with your chest up. This makes it difficult for the attacker to defend by pushing your head down or counterattack with a guillotine choke.

This takedown only requires you to catch one leg, and can work even if you fail to get your hips close to the attacker.

STARTING POSITION: Left-leg-forward fighting stance, facing the attacker.

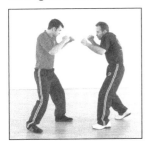

1. Drop low and shoot in quickly, wrapping your arms around one of the attacker's legs. We assume that you dropped very low, perhaps as if the attacker pushed you down, and that you catch his foot rather than his leg.

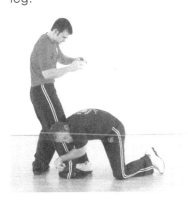

2–3. Pull his foot toward you and slightly upward while driving your shoulder into his shin just below his knee. Use your legs to help drive your shoulder. BE CAREFUL in training, because this takedown can damage the attacker's knee if done aggressively.

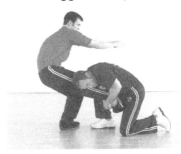

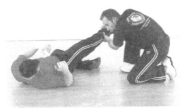

4. If you wish to continue attacking on the ground, move up to side mount. Otherwise, step back and stand up.

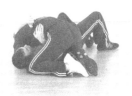

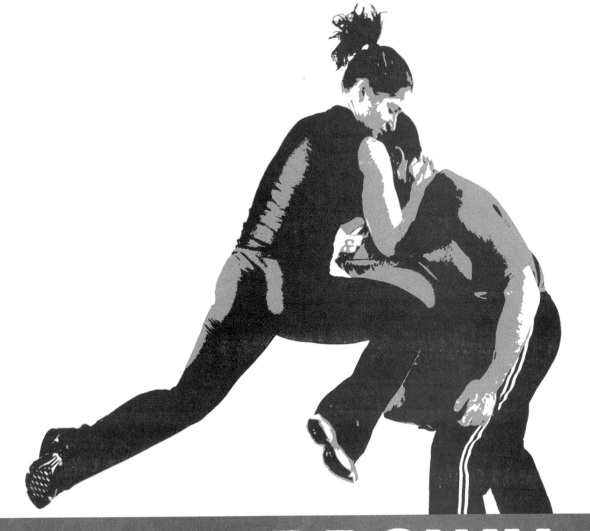

BROWN BELT

BROWN BELT

Brown Belt is the final level before the Black Belt test. At our Krav Maga Worldwide certified schools, you will sometimes see this listed as "Level 5," which denotes classes designed for Brown Belts, Black Belts, and above. At this level you will continue to learn to defend against guns, knives, and sticks. The angles of attack become harder to deal with, and the stress level increases, but because this is Krav Maga, the principles remain the same. In addition to handguns, in the firearms section we learn to deal with long guns such as shotguns and assault rifles. Expect to train at least 12 months at this level, assuming a minimum of two training sessions per week. By the end of Brown Belt training, you should feel that you can stand in the middle of a room, eyes closed, and be able to defend against any sort of attack: a bearhug, a choke, even an attack with a weapon.

COMBATIVES

The combative techniques described in the Brown Belt curriculum include more-advanced techniques, especially kicks that move beyond the fundamentals Krav Maga emphasizes. Among them are a number of kick combinations that include "switch kicks." Think of switch kicks in this way: the second kick is already en route as the first kick is recoiling. It is the switch that makes the kicks a true combination, rather than just one kick followed by another.

THROWS

Brown Belt introduces throws and holds not emphasized in earlier belt levels. In general, Krav Maga prefers to strike rather than throw, since in self-defense the defender is not responsible for taking the attacker into custody, nor necessarily in eliminating the attacker—only in eliminating the threat. Given this goal, a strike is often easier and more available than a throw. However, there are situations in which, due to balance or position, a throw may be the easiest way to reduce or eliminate the threat. You should understand that the main goal is to slam the attacker straight down to the ground, not to throw them far away.

DEFENSES

Brown Belt includes hand defenses against knife attacks, as well as advanced defenses against high-risk handgun threats and long gun threats.

EDGED-WEAPON DEFENSES

Although we teach a kick defense against knife attacks in Blue Belt, we assume that most often the attacker will surprise us, making hand defenses necessary. One prerequisite for understanding knife defenses is a basic understanding of commons ways to hold the knife. The three basic holds are regular (overhead) stab, underhand stab, and straight stab (page 218).

Very tight slashes can look a lot like straight stabs. Advanced training should include recognition of the angle of the knife hold. For example, if the arm is coming very straight toward the defender but the blade is angled outward, it is most likely a slash. This attack cannot be treated like a straight stab because the knife, angled out, prevents the defender from getting to the arm. By the same token, if the attacker keeps the point of the blade very much forward, even if he intends to slash, the defender can treat it as a straight stab. While disarms should be taught, real-life attacks and realistic training prove that they are not always possible. You should train to disengage at various points, such as:

1. Defend and counter, then disengage and look for common objects or other weapons;

2. Defend, counter, and deliver knees, then disengage and look for common objects or other weapons;

3. Defend, counter, deliver knees, get two hands on the weapon, then deliver more attacks.

A good understanding of state of readiness is vital to realistic knife-defense training. Once the technique is introduced and the basics have been mastered, you should learn to make the defense from varying states of readiness:

Very early: the defender is able to send the hands but also burst forward with the feet and defend the knife while it is back.

Moderately early: the defender is able to send the hands and get his weight very much forward, but there is minimal foot movement at the beginning.

Moderately late: the defender is able to send the hands forward and get some weight into the defense and counter, but with no footsteps at all.

Very late: the defender succeeds in making the 360° Defense and counterattacking, but without much forward shift of weight. In this case, the defender gets as much weight into the defense and counter as possible.

This last detail underscores an important element of Krav Maga training. All movements should cause the defender's weight to move forward so that, even in very late stages, you are in the habit of putting as much weight as possible into the defense and counterattack. From all states of readiness, the defender must move forward aggressively, regardless of his ability (or inability) to move his feet.

LEFT JAB/OVERHAND RIGHT COMBINATION

Combatives

The focus of this combination is the overhand right punch. An overhand punch belongs in the same family as a hook or an uppercut. All these punches are the same, just made on different planes.

STARTING POSITION: Left-leg-forward fighting stance.

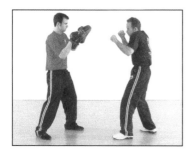

1. Deliver the left jab with an advance.

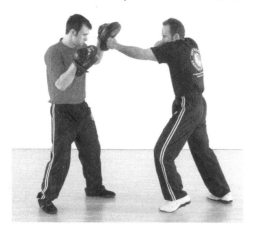

2. Send your right hand in a motion similar to a hook punch, but "turned over" so that your elbow is pointed up to the sky. Your right fist should also be turned over so that the pinky side is up and the thumb side, or "mouth" of the hand, is down. Make contact with the first two knuckles.

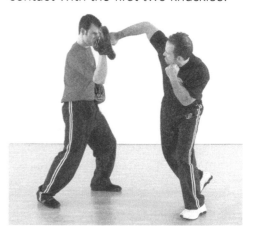

TIPS

Keep a bend in your elbow to get around (or over) a defense. However, the amount of bend in your elbow will depend on your distance from the target.

STARTING POSITION: Left-leg-forward fighting stance.

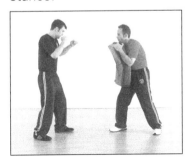

1. Deliver a front kick to a vertical target with your left foot.

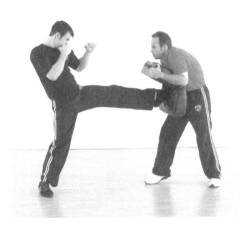

2–3. As the front kick makes contact, leap off your right foot. While in the air, tuck your left foot underneath you and deliver a round kick with your right foot. The kick should allow your hip to roll over.

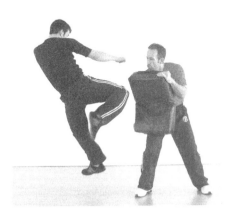

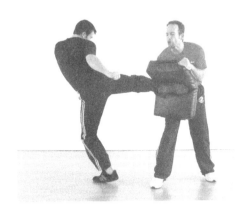

Bring both feet down into either a regular or opposite fighting stance, depending on your ability to recoil off the round kick.

TWO FRONT KICKS WITH A SWITCH

Combatives

STARTING POSITION: Left-leg-forward fighting stance.

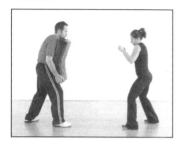

1. Deliver a front kick to a vertical target with your left foot.

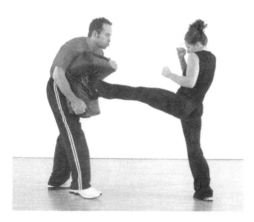

TIPS

It is sometimes preferable to begin this combination with your right foot forward.

2–3. As the first front kick lands, jump up with your right leg and deliver a second front kick. The first kick should be recoiling as the second kick lands.

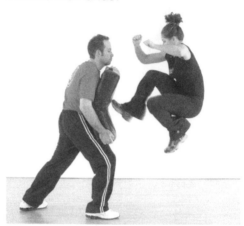

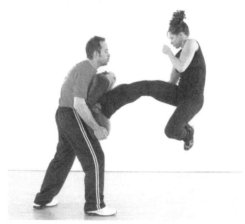

Bring both feet down into either a regular or opposite fighting stance.

STARTING POSITION: Left-leg-forward fighting stance.

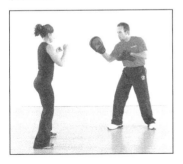

1. Make an outside slap kick with either leg.

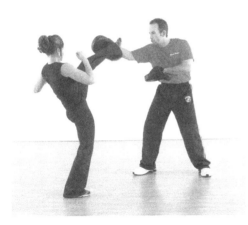

2–3. As the first kick begins to come down, deliver a front kick low to the groin.

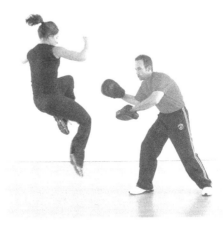

In this combination, you'll most likely end in an opposite fighting stance.

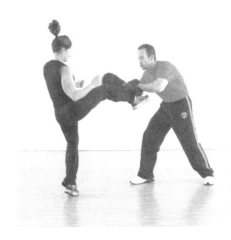

To hold for this combination, the holder should have two focus mitts (one held high for the slap kick, the other held low for the front kick). For safety reasons, the kicker should not make a strong front kick. If focus mitts are not available, use one small kicking shield for the front kick and, in this case, the kicker may have to make the slap kick to the air.

The outside slap kick is usually made relatively high.

TWO STRAIGHT KNEES WITH A SWITCH

Combatives

STARTING POSITION: Close to your opponent (while in a clinch or after a self-defense technique).

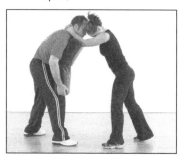

1. Grab and give a knee strike.

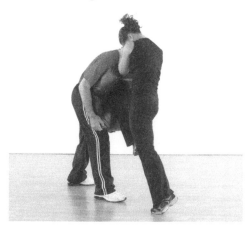

2. Immediately deliver the second knee just as the first knee is recoiling.

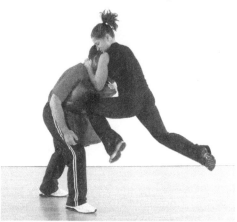

STARTING POSITION: Right-leg-forward fighting stance facing away from the target.

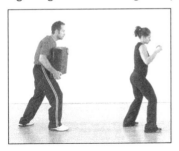

1. Deliver one back kick as usual.

2–3. As the first kick lands, immediately make a switch and deliver the second back kick. Your head should turn from one side to the other to allow for vision and balance in the second kick.

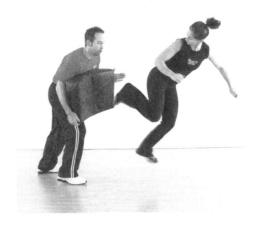

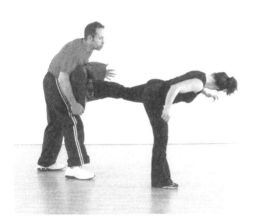

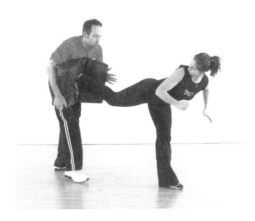

Throws

This takedown is so-named because it is useful against a threat with a submachine gun when the defender must move to the dead side. However, it is equally useful against handgun threats from the front or back when the defender is forced to the dead side and cannot control the weapon.

You must be aware that this technique does not effectively control the weapon. It is therefore high risk and should only be done when no other options are available.

STARTING POSITION: Facing the gunman; you are forced to move to his left side.[

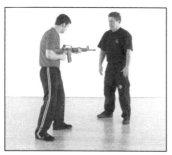

1. Redirect the weapon as in Long Gun from the Front—Dead Side (page 315).

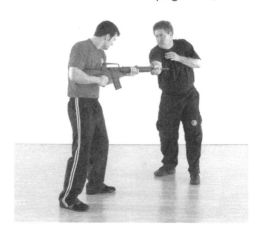

2. Burst in so that you are beside or slightly behind the gunman. Your hips must be close to him.

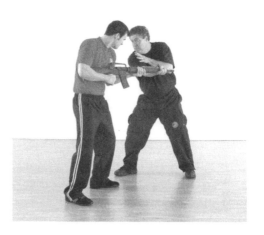

3. Your left hand should slide up and under the weapon, trapping it to his body. Your right hand reaches between his legs as far as possible (imagine trying to reach up and grab his belt buckle).

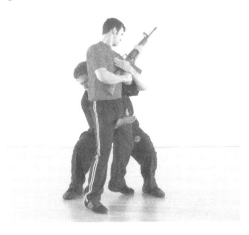

4. Use your legs (not your back) to lift him off his feet. As you lift, pull with your right arm so that his feet tilt up and his head tilts down.

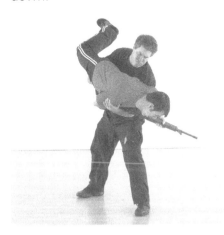

5. Drive him into the ground.

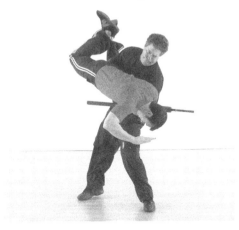

6. Land on him, delivering elbow strikes. If the weapon is out from under his body, be sure to control it.

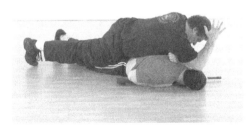

Additional beginning scenarios that can utilize this takedown defense when there is no other option: Gun from Behind, in Rear Hand, Forward Hand on Right Shoulder

Gun from the Front, in Rear Hand, Forward Hand Pushing/holding Center or Left Side

Throws

STARTING POSITION:
Attacker has made a
wide outside attack
similar to a haymaker;
you have defended and
counterattacked.

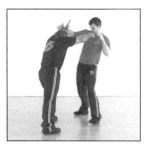

1. Grab the inside of the
attacker's wrist with your
left hand while stepping
in. As you step in, reach
your right arm under the
attacker's armpit. Your
goal is to get the crook of
your elbow in his armpit,
with your right forearm
reaching up. You should
also now have your back
to the attacker with your
hips square with his hips
and your own feet relatively
close together. Do NOT pull
his right arm or armpit up to
your shoulder/neck area.

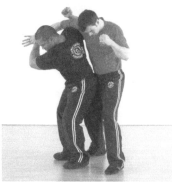

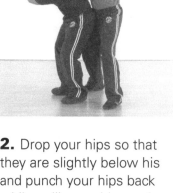

2. Drop your hips so that
they are slightly below his
and punch your hips back
while pulling on his arm/
shoulder. This should get the
attacker up on your back/
hips. When punching your
hips back, think of "low-
bridging" the attacker.

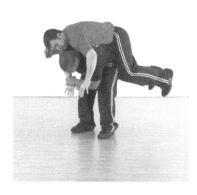

3–4. Continue to pull
forward while dropping
your right shoulder to your
left knee. This will take
the attacker over the top
and drop him down to the
ground.

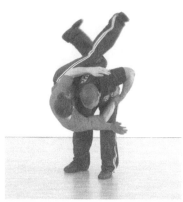

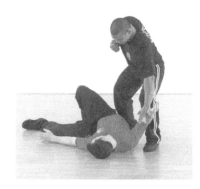

VARIATION: Instead of
reaching the crook of your
elbow under the attacker's
armpit, you can use your
right hand to grab his
shoulder or upper arm.

During the throw, you can
also try dropping low and
in while pulling the attacker
down. This causes him to
roll over the top of you. It
creates less impact when

he hits the ground, but is
possible when you cannot
get him up on your hips.

The hip roll is a variant of the one-arm shoulder throw. Instead of trapping the attacker's arm/shoulder, you grab him around the waist or neck.

STARTING POSITION:
Attacker has his right arm extended towards you, perhaps after making a wide hook that you have blocked.

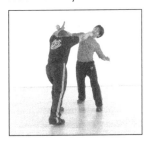

1. Grab the inside of the attacker's wrist with your left hand while stepping in. With your right arm, reach around the attacker's left hip. Ideally you'd grab at the belt or pants, but if nothing is available, grab skin or just wrap your hand/arm tightly around him. You should also now have your back to the attacker with your hips square with his hips and your own feet relatively close together. Drop your hips below his and punch them back, "lifting" him up onto your hips.

2–3. Using your arms for extra force, drive your right shoulder to your left hip, rolling him over the top of you and down into the ground.

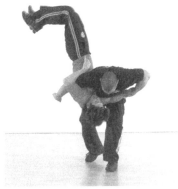

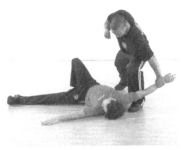

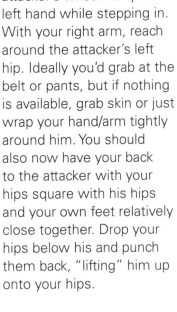

VARIATION: You can also wrap your right arm around the attacker's neck, rather than his waist, and grab at his shoulder.

FACE-TO-FACE FLIP ("SACRIFICE" THROW)

Throws

This throw is usually done successfully in a clinch when the attacker's weight is overcommitted forward. The attacker needs to know fall breaks, and you should have good mats on which to train.

STARTING POSITION: Left-leg-forward fighting stance.

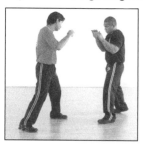

1–2. As the attacker comes in, grab his shirt collar tightly with both hands. Drop your weight down like you're sitting straight down toward the floor. Do NOT fall backward; you want to stay near the attacker. As you do so, bring your back foot up (with your knee bent tightly so it can fit between your body and your attacker's) and place it against the attacker's hip/belt buckle. It helps to center your foot on the attacker's body to avoid slipping off the hip, and to angle your foot with the heel in and toes pointed out.

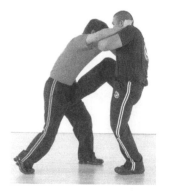

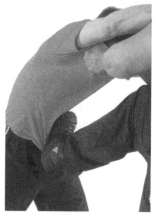

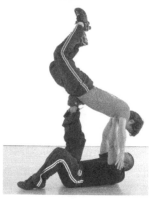

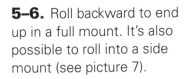

3–4. Round your back as you hit the floor. Continuing to hold on with your hands so that the attacker lands close to you, use your leg to kick/push the attacker over your head so that he flips and lands on his back.

5–6. Roll backward to end up in a full mount. It's also possible to roll into a side mount (see picture 7).

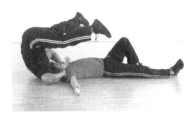

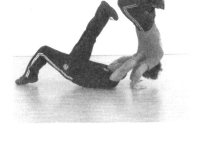

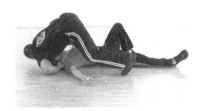

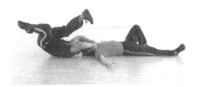

VARIATION: This can also be done in a clinch, with the attacker leaning his weight on you. It is also possible, although more difficult, to make the technique while doing a Muay Thai–style hold around the attacker's neck. Be sure you turn your head to one side to avoid an accidental headbutt.

Once you flip the attacker over, continue over in a somersault to land either in a full mount or side mount.

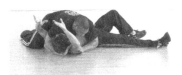

Self-Defense

This defense is made when the attacker jumps on the defender from behind and attempts to apply a headlock.

STARTING POSITION: The attacker jumps on you from behind and attempts to apply a headlock with his right arm.

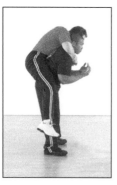

1. Tuck your chin and turn it to avoid the choke (in this example, the defender turns his chin to the left). Immediately drop your right shoulder to your left knee, rolling him over the top of you and straight down.

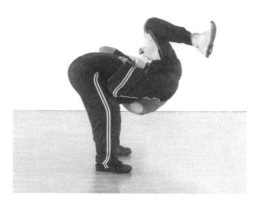

2. Continue with counters (punches, stomps, kicks, etc.).

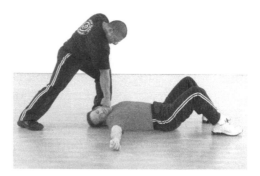

This defense is applied to a headlock from the side when the attacker tries to pull/spin the defender in and to the ground. This technique can also work against the static Yellow Belt headlock (page 68) when the attacker leans his weight far forward.

STARTING POSITION: Attacker applies a headlock from the side.

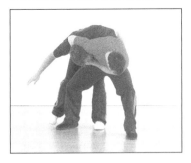

1. Go with the movement, tucking your chin in, swinging your outside hand to the groin, and bringing your inside arm up.

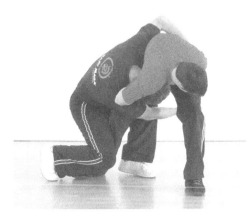

2. As you feel yourself being pulled farther in, swing your arm under his groin up to your shoulder (the goal is simply to make sure you are as close to him as possible). At the same time, continue taking your body close to him, with your inside leg very close to his body. Think of bringing your knee to the ground right between his feet. Your outside arm should have been coming up and will likely have grabbed the attacker's waist or shoulder.

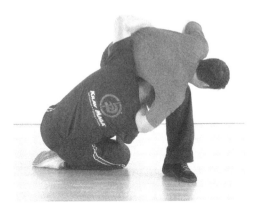

steps 3–5 continued on next page

Self-Defense

continued from previous page

3. Continue spinning in, using momentum as well as pulling with the hand grabbing the waist or shoulder, until you've pulled the attacker over your body and to the ground.

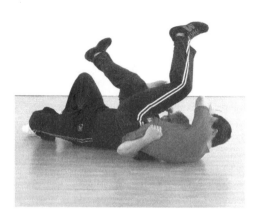

4. Roll to your knees beside him, using your free arm (the one that reached between his legs) to base out so he cannot roll you. This position is very similar to Headlock from the Side Defense—Attacker's Weight Back (page 205) in Green Belt.

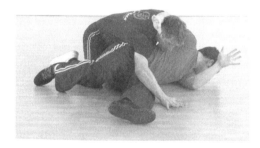

5. Deliver knee strikes, hammerfists, headbutts, etc., to counterattack.

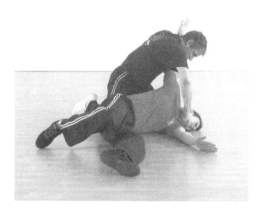

This defense is made against headlock attacks when the attacker gets a forearm under the defender's chin and tries to throw his (the attacker's) weight back, breaking the defender's neck. In most cases, tucking your chin in and down defends against this attack.

STARTING POSITION:

Attacker places his forearm under your chin in order to make a headlock from the side. You may have already initiated a headlock defense, bringing your outside hand up as though to grab his face.

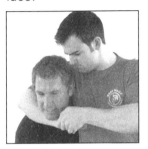

1. As you feel the attacker sit back, lifting your chin and creating pressure on your neck, immediately kick your inside foot forward, between his legs and into the air.

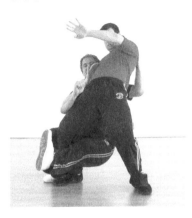

2. Drop your hips straight down to the ground and in hard while pulling with your left arm at his shoulder (or at his face, if you reached that high up in time). Be sure to keep your forearm pressed against his back in order to prevent your elbow from smashing into the ground.

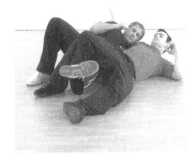

3. Continue with counterattacks such as punches, headbutts, and elbows.

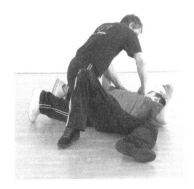

TIPS

If there is any impact on your arm during the takedown, it should occur along the length of your forearm, not your elbow.

DEFENSE AGAINST FULL NELSON: LEVERAGE ON THE FINGERS

Self-Defense

A full nelson is a hold in which the attacker, standing behind the defender, slides both arms under the defender's armpits, then up behind the defender's neck, clasping his hands together. The attack immobilizes the defender's arms and can put intense pressure on the defender's neck. Of the three defenses against full nelson, this is the easiest and is the one that should be tried first.

STARTING POSITION:
Attacker applies full nelson.

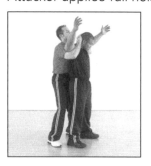

1–2. Immediately send both hands backward, stabbing at the attacker's eyes and face, then immediately strike, scratch, and claw at the attacker's hands at the back of your neck, prying at one of the fingers. Any finger will work, although the flexibility of the thumbs makes them less desirable. Try to grab the finger so that the index-finger side of your fist is near the base of the finger you grab.

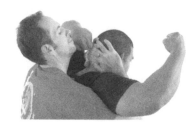

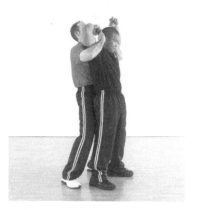

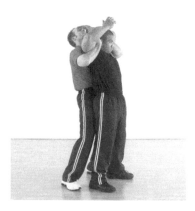

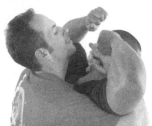

3. Strip that finger away to take the hand from your neck.

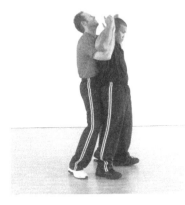

5. For added pressure, tuck your elbow in tight to your body, and lift.

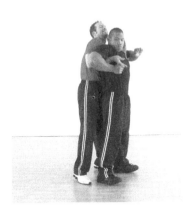

6. Step out to the same side as the hand you grabbed and deliver counterattacks with your free hand.

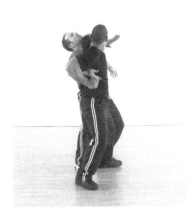

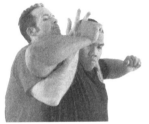

4. As the hand pulls away, bring your fist down and roll it in and up, bending the finger.

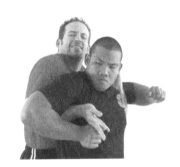

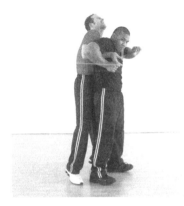

Self-Defense

This defense is usually applied when the fingers are not available, and should be performed if you feel you can shoot your hips back against the attacker.

STARTING POSITION: Attacker applies full nelson.

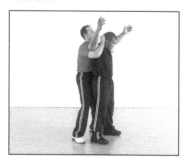

1. Bring your elbows down to try to loosen the attacker's grip.

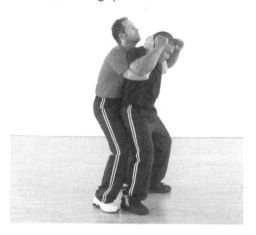

2. Drop your hips below the attacker's hips and punch them back, bringing the attacker up on your back.

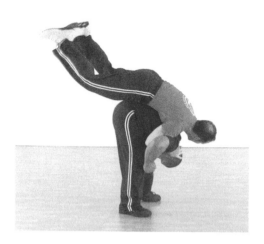

3. Drop one shoulder to the opposite knee and flip the attacker over you.

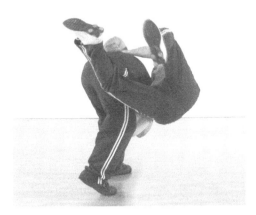

4. As he flips over, continue your spin so that you end up landing on top of him. Deliver counterattacks (elbows to the face, strikes to the groin).

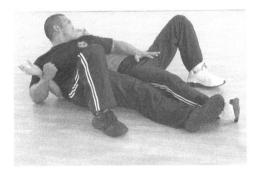

Self-Defense

This defense is usually applied when the fingers are not available, and should be performed if you feel that you can take a step with your foot.

STARTING POSITION: Attacker applies full nelson.

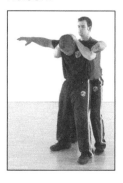

1. Clamp your elbows down—this might loosen the attacker's grip and also guarantees that he will now stay close.

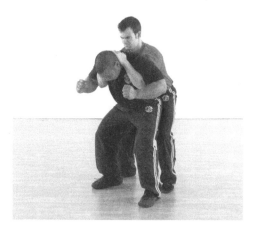

2–3. Shift your hips to one side and step back with your inside leg (i.e., if you shift your hips to the left, step back with your right foot), making sure your knee and foot are pointed in the same basic direction as the attacker's.

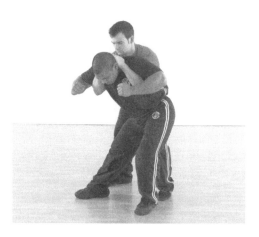

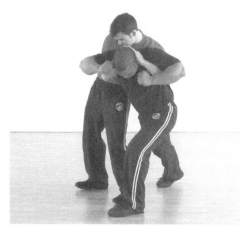

4. Sweep or punch your back leg forward. (If the attacker allows you to stand up tall, you can sweep; more often you will be crouched a little, in which case you should punch your knee forward). Your goal is to pop his leg forward, removing his base. At the same time, drive your upper body backward and down.

5–6. Land heavily on the attacker while delivering an elbow to the head. Continue with more counterattacks.

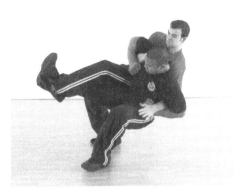

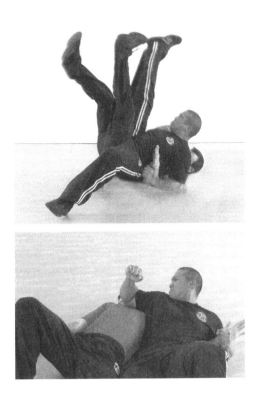

Knife Defenses

This is the most common type of knife attack, usually targeting the chest, clavicle, neck, and face.

STARTING POSITION: Modified passive stance.

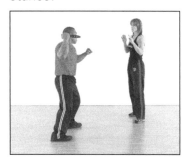

1. As the attacker bursts forward, use the 360° Defense to attack the knife hand and strike the attacker. The defense should be made wrist to wrist. Think of attacking the attack with your defense. Also, think of punching with full power!

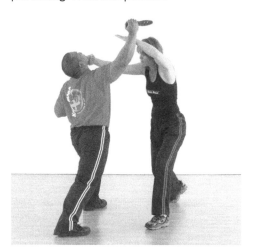

2. Continue to burst forward, driving the attacker's arm back and down while rotating your wrist in to catch his wrist in your hand. Be sure to keep your weight back and down on his arm. This will make it difficult for him to recoil and stab again.

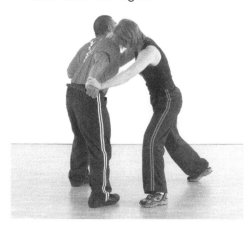

3. With your inside arm braced against his body (elbow down, forearm against neck), deliver knees explosively.

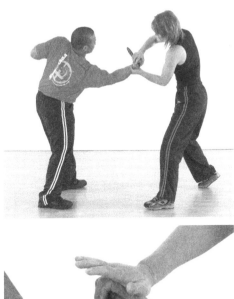

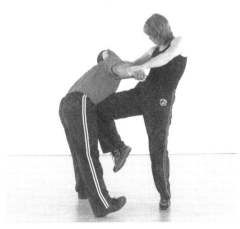

4–5. Only attempt a disarm if you have sufficiently softened the attacker and have good control. To disarm, bring his knife hand inward and cap it with your right hand.

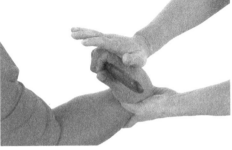

steps 6–7 continued on next page

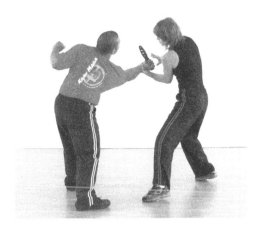

Knife Defenses

continued from previous page

6–7. Make a cavalier and strip the knife.

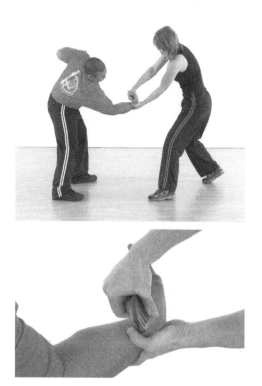

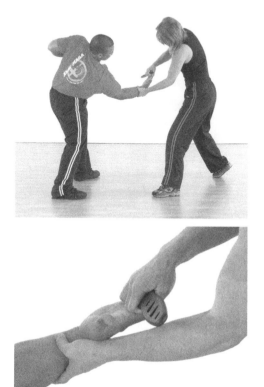

TIPS
If you encounter resistance while attempting the disarm, deliver kicks to the groin, headbutts, etc.

Another common attack is the upward stab, either vertical or at a diagonal angle. Note that the technique described first assumes that the stab is made upward, but at a slight inward angle, from outside the attacker's body up and in. This is the most common and natural form of the attack.

STARTING POSITION: Modified passive stance.

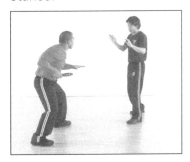

1. Attacker stabs upward, at a slight inward angle, from outside the attacker's body up and in. As the attacker bursts forward, use the 360° Defense (#6 or #7) to attack the knife hand and strike the attacker. The defense must be made wrist to wrist (if not, the stab will come up and underneath the defense). Think of attacking the attack with your defense. Also, think of punching with full power!

2. Immediately push his arm outward and backward with your forearm, then reach your arm out in a motion very similar to Gun from Behind (page 253). Bring your arm in sharply to trap the knife hand at your chest/ shoulder exactly like Gun from Behind.

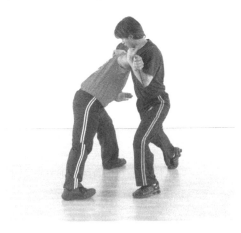

steps 3–8 continued on next page

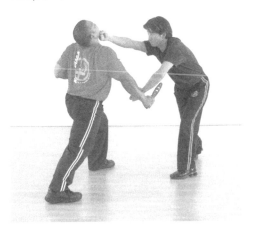

Knife Defenses

continued from previous page

3. Deliver knees or groin kicks explosively, keeping your weight forward and on the attacker.

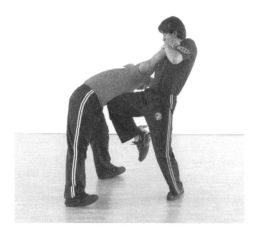

4. Keeping the arm trapped, reach your right hand over and "cover" the knife hand (your hand and fingers should point the same direction as the attacker's).

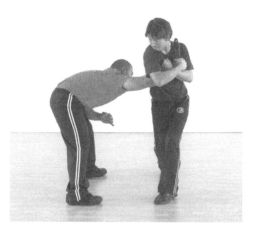

5. Rotate his wrist sharply so that the pinky side of his hand is toward the ceiling.

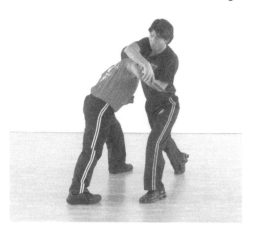

6–7. Turn your left shoulder toward the attacker, putting pressure on his wrist and arm. Quickly release your trapping hand (left) and slide it down to grab his wrist. As you do, step out a little bit, but keep weight on his arm and wrist.

8. Make a cavalier and strip the knife from his hand.

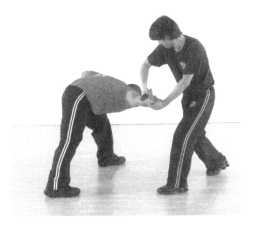

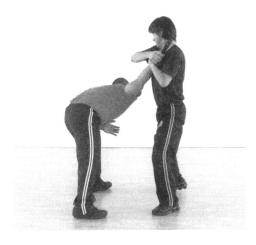

If you meet resistance, kick to the face or groin.

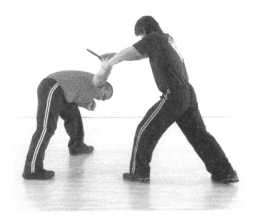

VERTICAL UPWARD STAB VARIATION: In some cases, the attacker stabs in a vertical motion up the middle of the attacker's body. In this case, the initial defense is exactly the same. However, the control is different because the nature of the attack does not allow the defender to push the attacking arm outward.

Once the defense is made, if the defender finds himself more on the dead side, the defender should make the control and disarm used in Defense against Straight Stab (page 304).

KNIFE DEFENSE AGAINST STRAIGHT STAB

Knife Defenses

Straight stabs are less common than upward or downward stabs. However, they can be done and must be defended. There is a hold specific to straight stab wherein the pommel (butt end) of the knife is pressed into the palm of the attacker's hand. However, this hold is less secure and not always used by attackers. Most often, they will hold the knife in a regular grip (blade upward). In this case, the only indication the attacker may give you of his intention to make a straight stab is to stand with the knife-side leg forward.

STARTING POSITION: Left-leg-forward fighting stance as attacker makes right-handed stab.

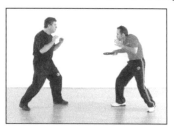

1. Redirect the attack using your left hand, rotating your hand sharply ("chop") against the back of the attacker's hand to increase the movement away from your body.

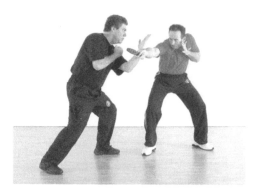

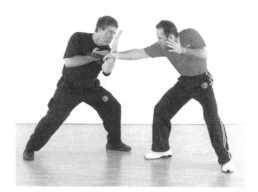

2. Burst forward at a slight angle, sliding your arm forward and reaching down to catch the attacker's arm. Be sure your elbow stays down to prevent the attacker from slashing, and be sure you keep weight forward on the arm to make the attacker feel jammed. At the same time, deliver a strong right punch.

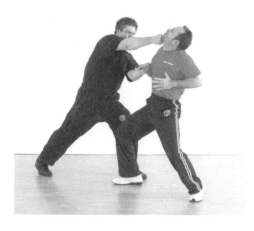

3–6. As you recoil your punch, bring your right hand down and cover the attacker's hand. Continue to put weight forward toward the attacker. Make a cavalier and strip the knife, kicking to the groin if necessary.

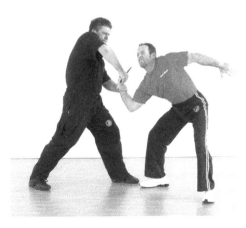

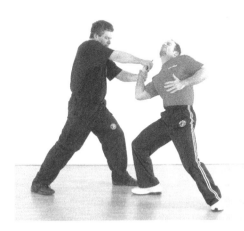

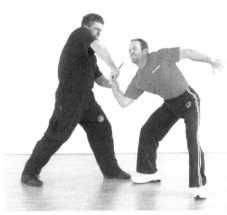

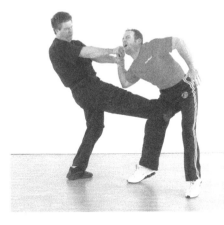

If you feel resistance, you can make another cavalier with a takedown.

TIPS

Since we are usually a little late in defending, a general guideline is: "If you aim for the knife you'll get the hand." Because this defense is slightly more difficult, we recommend that you begin training from a fighting stance. Once you have mastered the technique, train from a passive stance as well.

KNIFE DEFENSE AGAINST STRAIGHT STAB (LIVE SIDE)

Knife Defenses

It may be necessary to defend a straight stab to the live side, most commonly because the attacker is left-handed. Since we train so often against right-handed attacks, it is unrealistic to ask defenders to recognize the left-handed attack and make the defense from the opposite side. However, it might also be a right-handed attack that comes from the right side. The descriptions here will assume the first example, which is most common.

STARTING POSITION: Left-leg-forward fighting stance as attacker makes left-handed stab.

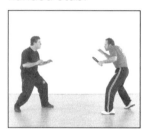

1. Redirect the attack using your left hand, rotating your hand sharply ("chop") against the inside of the attacker's hand to increase the movement away from your body. More emphasis should be placed on a larger hand and body defense because of the possibility of a bend in the attacker's elbow. As you defend, keep your right hand close to your body to avoid the redirected knife.

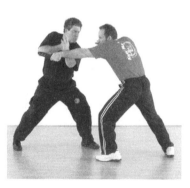

2. Immediately send a chop or hammerfist to the attacker's neck or face while simultaneously sending your right hand toward the attacker's bicep to catch the arm. Go to the bicep because you know where that part of the arm will be—if you reach for the wrist, it will be recoiling away from you and harder to catch.

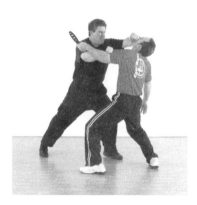

3. Put weight on the attacker, exploding in with knees or groin kicks. Try to get the forearm of your right hand against the attacker's knife arm in a way that makes it difficult for him to stab, but attack aggressively regardless of arm position. Slide your hand down to catch his wrist and deliver more knee strikes.

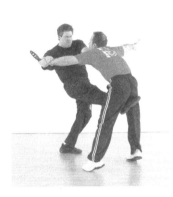

4–6. When the attacker is softened, bring his knife hand inward and cap it with your right hand. Make a cavalier and strip the knife.

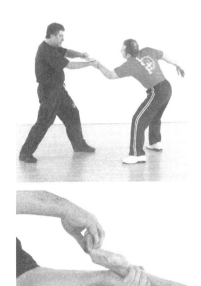

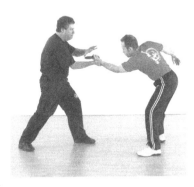

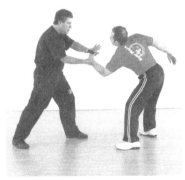

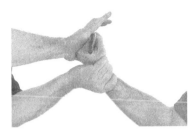

TIPS

The only difference between this disarm and the disarm in Defense against Downward Stab (page 298) is that, because of the nature of the knife grip, the blade will be closer to your arm and body. Be sure to keep the knife close to him and far from you.

KNIFE DEFENSE AGAINST FORWARD SLASH

Knife Defenses

The Defense against Forward Slash is almost exactly like 360° with Counterattack (page 112). The only difference is that, if you see the knife coming, you should get your head inside and tuck your chin to avoid the knife accidentally "flicking" or flying into your face or neck as you defend.

STARTING POSITION: Passive stance as attacker makes right-handed forward slash.

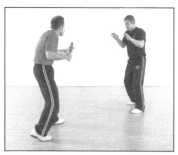

1. Make a 360° Defense against his wrist as you make a right punch to his face. Tuck your chin down and get your head inside the defense to avoid the knife.

2–3. Push the knife arm back and down, catch at the wrist, and deliver knees.

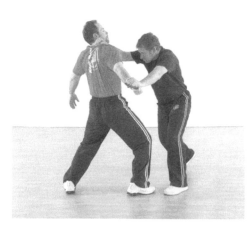

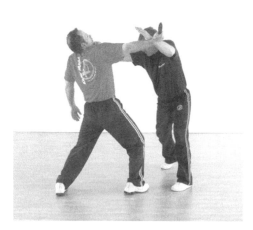

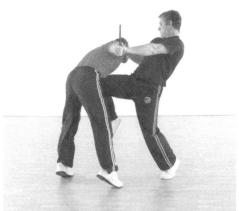

4. To disarm, bring his knife hand inward
and cap it with your right hand.

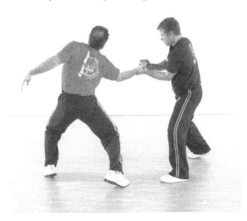

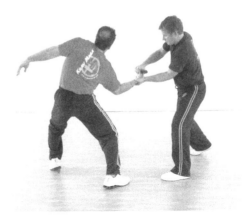

5–7. Make a cavalier and strip the knife. Be
aware that the knife blade is pointing toward
you, so make sure to bring the knife in and
close to the attacker, not close to you.

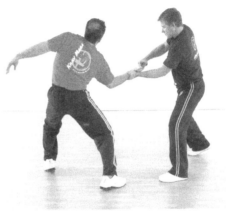

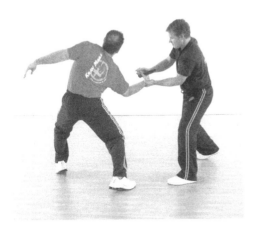

Knife Defenses

STARTING POSITION:
Modified passive stance
facing the attacker.

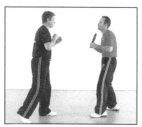

1. As the attacker makes
a forward slash, lean back
and away (this may happen
reflexively).

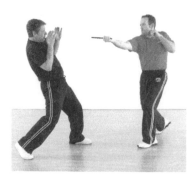

2. Immediately burst back
into the fight. Block the
attack with both forearms—
one above and one below
the attacking elbow. Keep
your chin tucked and try to
lean your head and body
inward toward the attacker.

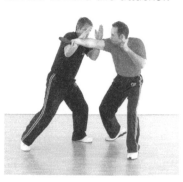

3–4. Pivot your forward
arm (usually your left hand
against a right-handed slash)
down to catch close to the
attacker's wrist, then punch
with your rear hand (usually
your right). Note that this
position is exactly like the
control and counterattack
position used in Defense
against Straight Stab (page
304).

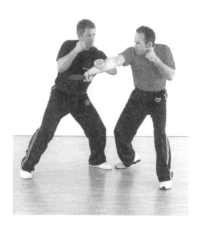

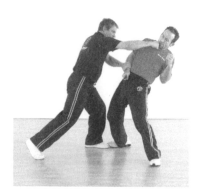

5. To disarm, bring his knife hand inward and cap it with your right hand.

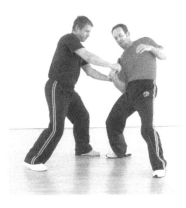

6–7. Make a cavalier and strip the knife.

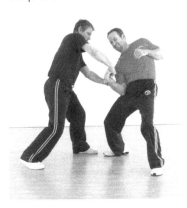

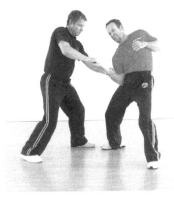

Shotgun/Assault Rifle/Submachine Gun Defenses

STARTING POSITION: Passive stance.

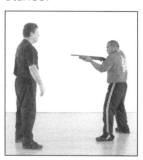

1. As the attacker presents the rifle, send your left hand to the weapon in a straight line, keeping your hand open and your fingers extended downward at about a 45-degree angle. Keeping your left arm stiff, put the palm of your hand at the barrel of the weapon and push in a straight line to your right. As you redirect, make a body defense by allowing your left shoulder to come forward and blading (or turning) your body; this has the added benefit of putting your motion and weight toward the gunman even though your feet have not yet moved. Your left hand should move first, but as it does, your right hand should then move inward to avoid the line of fire. Think of moving the right hand to the crook of the left elbow.

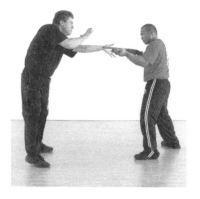

2. Burst forward with your feet toward the rifleman, sliding your left hand toward the butt while your right hand replaces the left. ALWAYS maintain contact with the weapon.

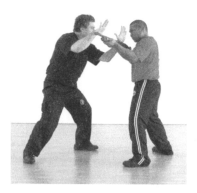

3. Grab the weapon sharply with both hands, keeping your elbows down to maintain control. Be sure your left hand has gone deep to defend against or prevent a strike with the butt end. You should already be putting weight on the weapon, driving it toward the attacker.

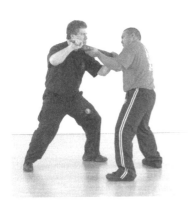

4. With a firm grasp on the rifle, deliver a kick to the rifleman's groin area with either leg. Since your left leg will be closest to the rifleman, a kick delivered with this leg will get to the target sooner but won't have as much power as a kick delivered with the right leg, which will take slightly longer to reach the target. If you kick with your rear leg, be sure your weight is distributed forward. If you lean back while kicking with the rear leg, you may be shoved backward.

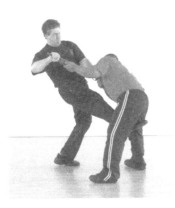

5. After you kick, plant your feet and sharply jerk the weapon upward so the muzzle rises. This will not release the hold, but generally puts the weapon in a better position for you.

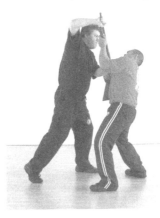

steps 6–8 continued on next page

continued from previous page

6. Immediately pull your left hand a little toward your body while your right hand, near the muzzle, punches the barrel towards the rifleman's face (similar to an overhand right punch).

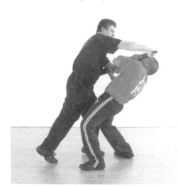

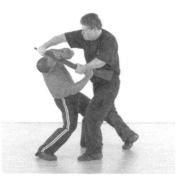

7–8. Recoil slightly, then drive the muzzle sharply past the rifleman's right shoulder and down to "break" it from his grasp. As soon as you are sure the weapon is in your possession, retreat to a

safe distance. Be prepared to use the rifle as a cold weapon.

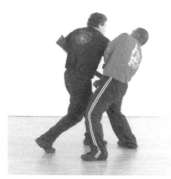

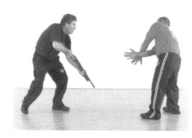

TIPS

The redirecting movement should take the rifle off your body parallel to the floor. Any diagonal movement up or down means that the rifle stays on your body for a longer period of time. This initial redirection must be a "punch" with your hand because the rifleman will have both hands on the weapon, which gives him greater control.

Note these differences when dealing with an assault weapon with a long magazine or handle attached, as opposed to a shotgun or rifle:

Because of the bottom-feeding magazines attached to most assault weapons, you may need to raise the weapon before delivering any type of kick, or else the magazine may block your leg as you attempt to kick the suspect's groin.

1. After delivering the counterattack kicks, use your left hand to lift the top of the assault weapon and pull the butt out from under the gunman's armpit.

2. Push the rear of the weapon down and over the top of the gunman's wrist in order break his hold.]

3. Then drive the barrel toward the gunman's face (similar to an overhead right punch).

Shotgun/Assault Rifle/Submachine Gun Defenses

STARTING POSITION: Passive stance.

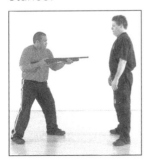

1. As the attacker presents the rifle, send your right hand to the weapon in a straight line, keeping your hand open and your fingers pointing towards the ground at a 45° angle. Keeping your right arm stiff, put the palm of your hand at the barrel of the weapon and push in a straight line to your left. This has the added benefit of putting your motion and weight toward the gunman even though your feet have not yet moved. Your right hand should move first, but after it begins, bring your left hand to the crook of your right elbow to keep it out of the line of fire.

2. Burst forward and to the right with your feet to the "dead side" of the rifleman and grab the weapon sharply with your left hand. Keep your arm straight to control the barrel and stay out of the line of fire. You should already be putting weight down and away on the weapon.

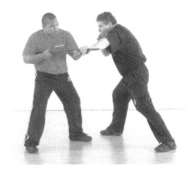

steps 3–8 continued on next page

Shotgun/Assault Rifle/Submachine Gun Defenses

continued from previous page

3–4. With a firm grip on the barrel, deliver a kick to the rifleman's groin area with your left leg. As you recoil your kick, jerk on the weapon to begin to loosen it as you deliver an overhand right punch to the head.

5–6. After your punch, recoil your right hand to reach under the rifleman's left arm and grasp the rifle, then pull the weapon upward slightly.

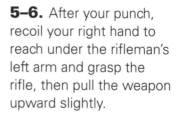

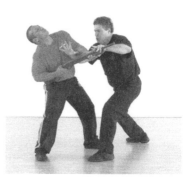

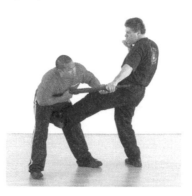

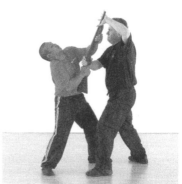

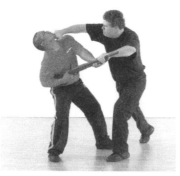

7. Take the left hand that is gripping the barrel and drive the barrel towards the rifleman's face (similar to an overhand left punch).

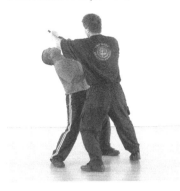

8. Rotate the rifle sharply past the rifleman's right shoulder to "break" his grasp. If the rifleman continues to hold onto the weapon, continue to strike him with the rifle, including kicks, knees, and headbutts, to soften his grip. As soon as you are sure the weapon is in your position, retreat to a safe distance. Be prepared to use the rifle as a cold weapon.

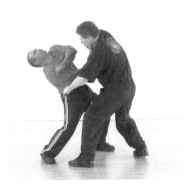

The redirecting movement should take the rifle off your body parallel to the floor. Any diagonal movement up or down means that the rifle stays on your body for a longer period of time. This initial redirection must be a "punch" with your hand because the rifleman will have both hands on the weapon, which gives him greater control.

It is unlikely that the control and disarm portions of this defense will be successful against a submachine gun. Sub guns simply offer very little surface to control on the dead side. This is exactly why Machine Gun Takedown (page 282) was created.

variation continued on next page

Shotgun/Assault Rifle/Submachine Gun Defenses

continued from previous page

DISARMING OVER GUNMAN'S LEFT ARM VARIATION: This variation of the "dead side" disarm is necessary if the gunman has clamped his left elbow down, preventing you from coming under his arm. The redirection, control, and counterattack for disarming from "under or over" the rifleman's arm are the same.

1. After you punch the rifleman with your right fist, recoil your right hand and reach over the rifleman's left arm and grasp the rifle towards the rear of the weapon.

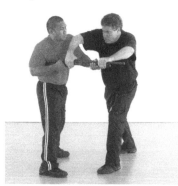

2. Push down and away with your right hand in order to clear the butt of the rifle from under the rifleman's right armpit. You should twist both wrists as though revving a motorcycle engine—this twists the weapon out and away from the gunman's grip.

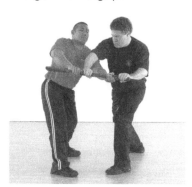

3–4. Pull the stock of the weapon up, striking the rifleman's face, and continue through with this movement, bringing the rifle to your body.

5–7. Take the left hand that is gripping the barrel and drive the barrel toward the rifleman's face (similar to an overhand left punch). rotating the rifle sharply past the rifleman's left shoulder to "break" his grasp.

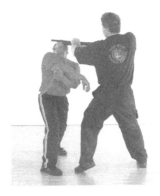

If the rifleman continues to hold onto the weapon, continue to strike him with the rifle and combatives to soften his grip.

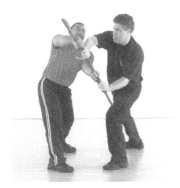

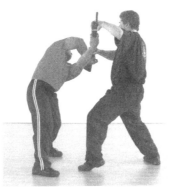

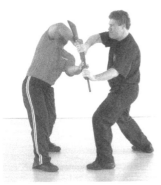

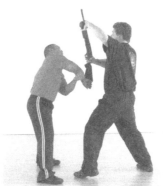

LONG GUN FROM THE SIDE, BEHIND THE ARM

Shotgun/Assault Rifle/Submachine Gun Defenses

The initial movements for this technique are very similar to Gun from the Side, Behind the Arm (page 248).

STARTING POSITION: Passive stance.

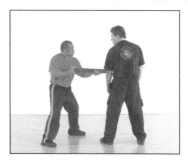

1. As the attacker places the rifle behind your arm, make a small redirection with your arm, pushing the rifle off line behind you. This movement should be relatively small.

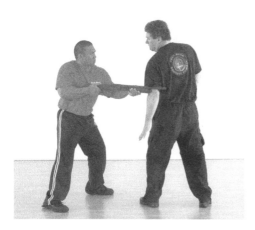

2. Turn toward the rifleman, reaching toward him with your inside hand (the one that made the redirection) so that your arm slips underneath his. Your goal should be to reach as deep as possible even before you've moved your feet. Burst in very deep so that your forward foot is outside the attacker's.

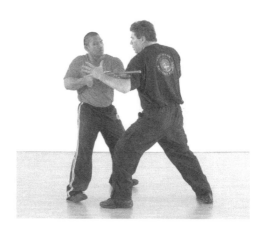

3. Wrap your forward arm up, bringing your hand and fingers up and over the top of the rifle, tightly trapping the barrel in the bend of your elbow. Unlike with a handgun, do not make a fist. A fist will not make the same hold on the rifle.

5. Take your shoulder on the weapon side and push it forward, forcing the barrel up, then slide your hand up and grab the barrel. You can skip the shoulder movement and go straight for the grab if you feel that he is not holding on firmly.

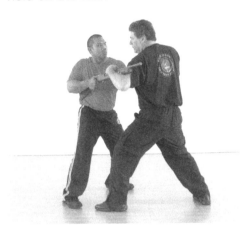

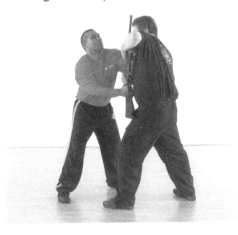

4. With your rear arm, deliver an elbow strike or overhead right punch to the gunman's face. Follow with knees if necessary.

steps 6–9 continued on next page

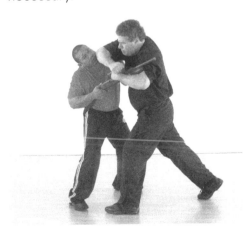

Shotgun/Assault Rifle/Submachine Gun Defenses

continued from previous page

6–7. Take your left hand that is gripping the barrel and drive the barrel towards the rifleman's face (similar to an overhand punch). At the same time, pull the butt of the rifle in your right hand to your right hip.

8–9. Rotate the barrel sharply past the rifleman's right shoulder to "break" it from his grasp. If the rifleman continues to hold onto the weapon, continue to strike him with the rifle and combatives to soften his grip.

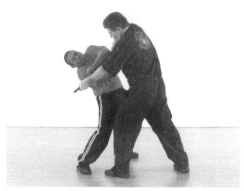

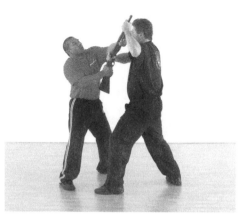

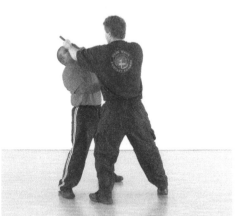

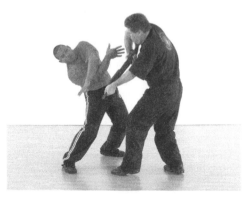

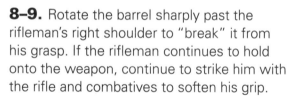

How the attacker presents the weapon (holding it with his right or left side forward) will determine which shoulder you rotate the barrel past on the disarm. If the long gun is presented on your right side, the same technique works, but in a mirror image, of course!

The technique for Long Gun from Behind is exactly the same as Long Gun from the Side, Behind the Arm (page 320), with a couple of small differences.

STARTING POSITION: Passive stance.

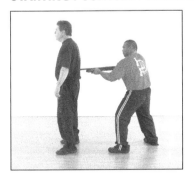

1. As the attacker touches the rifle to your back, look behind you. You aren't really concerned about what is touching your body—you need to make sure what type of weapon the attacker has in his possession.

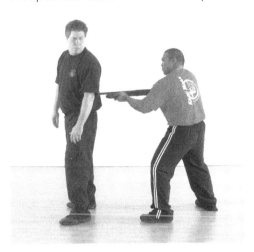

2. Leading with your arm, turn deeply enough to redirect the weapon and take your body out of the line of fire. Your body defense should cause you to immediately lean back (toward the attacker) even before your feet move.

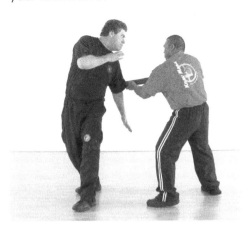

The control, counterattack, and disarm is the same as Long Gun from the Side, Behind the Arm.

TIPS

If the rifle is held low, your arm will make the redirection along with the body defense. If the rifle is held high on your back, your arm will have little or no effect, and you'll mostly make a body defense. However, the arm still helps your body rotate.

Shotgun/Assault Rifle/Submachine Gun Defenses

The Defense against Rifle/Bayonet Stab to the Live Side is exactly like the Defense against Long Gun from the Front—Live Side (page 312). The only significant differences are: 1) with a bayonet stab we are less concerned with telegraphing movement while in the line of fire; and 2) we must reach past the blade to defend along the barrel.

STARTING POSITION: Passive stance.

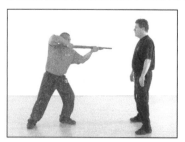

1. As your left hand makes the defense, lean forward so that you can reach past the blade.

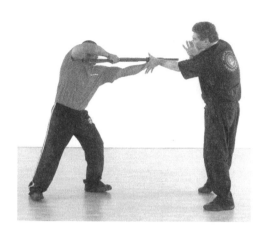

Shotgun/Assault Rifle/Submachine Gun Defenses

As with the defense to the live side, the initial defense is almost exactly like the Defense against Long Gun from the Front—Dead Side (page 316). The considerations here are the same as those for defense to the live side (leaning forward to reach past the cutting edge).

STARTING POSITION: Passive stance.

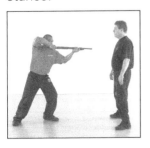

1–2. After the redirection is made with your right hand, sweep your right hand across his face to lift his chin (beneficial in military applications against opponents wearing helmets). With your left arm, deliver a "clothesline" with your left arm and step past the attacker with your left foot.

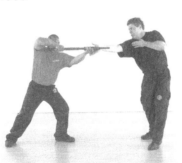

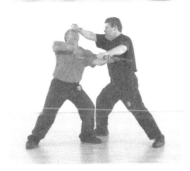

3–4. Drag the attacker up on your hip and "hang" him there, or take him down with a hip roll.

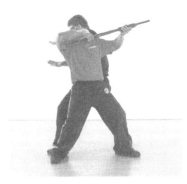

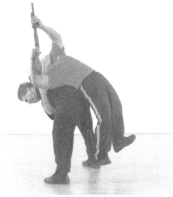

It is more difficult to execute this takedown on the live side because the attacker's hip is back, making it harder to step past that hip for the takedown.

DEFENSE AGAINST THREAT WITH A HANDGUN: FROM BEHIND AT A DISTANCE

Handgun Defenses

This threat represents a difficult situation for the defender—not because the movement is difficult, but because it is often difficult to gauge depth when glancing behind you. We say "From Behind at a Distance" to distinguish from Gun from Behind, Touching, which we presented in Blue Belt. Keep in mind that "distance" must still mean "within reach."

STARTING POSITION: Neutral stance.

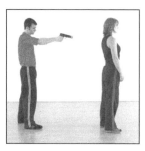

1. As the attacker makes the threat with his right hand, glance over your shoulder—do NOT make the move too aggressive.

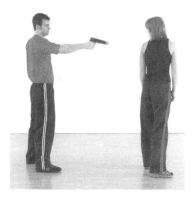

2. Using the hand on the same side you have looked, send that hand backward in a straight line to the weapon. Be sure your hand goes straight up and back, and that it does NOT arc out to the side and up. Think of the same principles as Gun from the Front (page 244). As your hand moves up, keep your thumb hooked to increase your chances of making contact with the gun. As your hand reaches the gun and redirects it to the side, make a body defense by turning your shoulder in toward the gun.

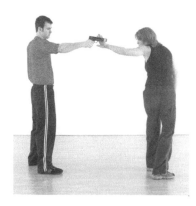

3. Burst toward the attacker, pushing the weapon back as you punch with your free hand.

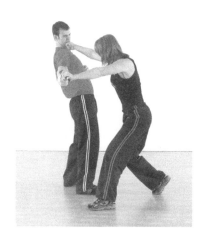

4. Recoil your punch and catch the attacker's wrist. Be sure you keep your weight on the weapon as you deliver kicks, headbutt, or knee strikes.

5. To disarm, continue pushing the muzzle forward while pulling at the wrist. This will snap the weapon and loosen his grip.

6. Pull the weapon down at an angle and retreat. Be sure you do NOT roll the weapon straight down, or the muzzle will point at your legs.

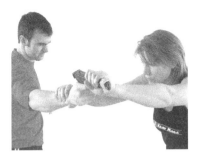
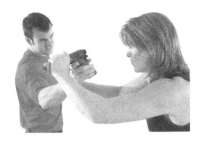
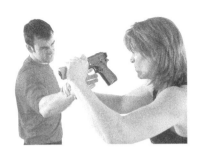

VARIATION: It is possible to make the redirection and catch the wrist immediately, skipping the punch. The advantage of this is that you secure the weapon more quickly. However, your counterattack takes longer, giving the attacker more time to fight against you.

A Note Regarding the Live Side and Dead Side: This technique works equally well whether you end up on the attacker's live side or dead side. If you make the defense to the attacker's dead side, you will usually end up driving the weapon inward to his body. Be aware that there is some danger of the attacker turning so that his back is to you. Be prepared to move your feet! If you make the defense to the attacker's live side, the attacker's arm has range of motion (his body is not in the way). Be sure you drive the weapon back aggressively, or you will end up "chasing" the weapon as his arm moves into the open space.

DEFENSE AGAINST THREAT WITH A HANDGUN: "CUPPING" TECHNIQUE (TWO HANDS)

Handgun Defenses

This technique can be used against threats from the front at any height, or to the side of the head. In threats from the front, it is used when the line of fire is placed offline, or when the defender does not want to redirect the weapon toward third parties. It is also used when the defender moves the line of fire and finds himself on the attacker's live side. In gun to the side of the head, it is used when the defender redirects the line of fire and finds himself on the attacker's live side.

STARTING POSITION: Neutral stance. The right-handed gunman points the weapon left of center on your body.

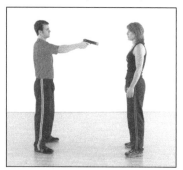

1. Using your right hand, redirect the weapon off to your left side. All the details regarding movement in Gun from the Front (page 244) apply.

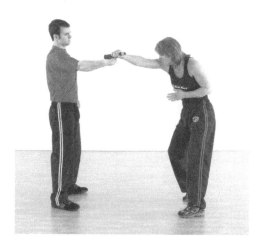

2. Immediately reach your left hand underneath and catch the gun at the back of the slide or hammer area. Your weight should already be transitioning forward. Burst forward diagonally with your left foot, keeping weight down and forward on the weapon. Simultaneously deliver a right front kick to the groin. Be sure your chin is down and your inside (right) shoulder is up to protect against a punch.

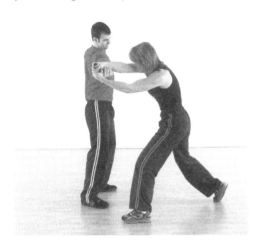

3–4. Disarm using the same movements used in Gun from the Front.

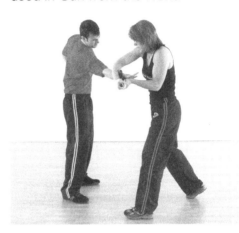

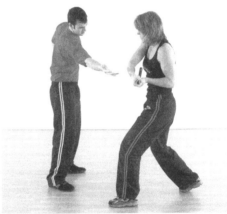

TIPS

In the initial position, it would not make sense to do regular Defense against Gun from the Front because the line of fire would track across the defender's entire body. (Alternately, imagine the gun pointed directly at the center of your chest; however, there is someone to your right, preventing you from making the regular defense.)

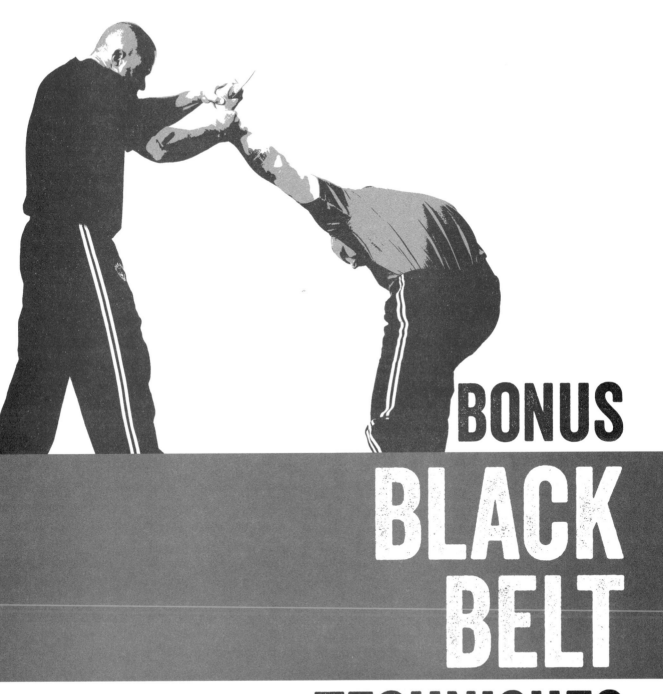

BONUS BLACK BELT TECHNIQUES

BONUS BLACK BELT TECHNIQUES

This chapter covers some advanced techniques that address a small selection of handgun and edged-weapon threats. It's a very small sampling from Krav Maga Worldwide's carefully designed and vastly evolved Black Belt Level curriculum. Needless to say, the topics presented are extremely high risk and involve the potential use of deadly force. Some exercises will be based more on principle than technique, taking into account the many variables that may affect intricate technical responses. *Note:* This chapter was not written in an effort to replace training with an updated and presently certified Krav Maga Worldwide instructor. Rather, the information is meant to serve as a resource for advanced instructors and an introduction for other instructors and students wishing to further their knowledge in the system. It bears repeating that the scenarios presented in this book are of extreme high risk, and no medium can replace actual supervised training.

USE OF FORCE: THE RULES OF SELF-DEFENSE

If you are reading this book, especially this chapter, it is safe to assume that you have an interest in developing your ability to defend yourself. If you are physically attacked as a target of an aggravated assault, a rape, an attempted murder or some other violent crime, having the

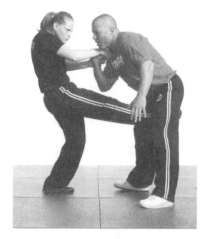

physical and tactical skills to survive the encounter may truly be a matter of life and death.

Self-defense instructors often teach their students to win at all costs—to do anything and everything to survive, to punish the assailant for assaulting you. Some may believe these statements to be true; however, such advice is usually proclaimed out of context and may have significant, negative, long-term, life-changing ramifications that involve legal battles in both civil and criminal arenas. You should be familiar with use of force law and its effect on your right to use self-defense, even deadly force, should the need arise. You must be prepared to win the battle on the street, while conducting yourself lawfully and ethically so that you survive the legal battles that may follow in the courts. Bottom line: know the law in your state! Here are some things to keep in mind:

Retreat Rule: If you *know* you can retreat without risking injury, you must do so.

"True Man" Doctrine: If you did not initiate the encounter, you are not obligated to retreat (so long as your assailant still poses a threat) even if you can do so safely.

Castle Doctrine: An exception to the retreat rule: If you are in your own home, you are not obligated to retreat, even under a state following the retreat rule.

Peterson Doctrine: If you're the initial aggressor you can't use self-defense as a justification for a use of force, unless you've made a good-faith showing that you wanted to stop fighting.

If you do get into a situation that escalates into a physical altercation, follow these after-action suggestions:

- Contact the police and your legal counsel as soon as possible.

- If you or the assailant are injured, obtain medical treatment by notifying the proper authorities.

- If available, obtain witness statements. The use of audio recording is strongly recommended to preserve witness statements and to prevent a change in a witness's testimony at a later date.

- Obtain the names and address of all individuals present and document their observations or lack of observations.

- If you have pain or visible injury, use a camera, whenever possible, to photograph the injured area. The photographs of the area should be before and after treatment by medical personnel. The post-medical treatment photograph should show the area without the bandage or covering, or if you have disheveled and torn clothing, this should also be photographed.

- If the aggressor complains of pain or has visible injury, summon the required medical treatment and even apply first aid if safe and necessary to do so.

HANDGUNS

The handguns section deals with a selection of extreme, high-risk scenarios in which an assailant, armed with a handgun, poses an imminent threat to the life of the defender under intense conditions. As variables increase, difficulties analyzing and reacting to the threats also increase. The Krav Maga principles applied to addressing threats and attacks are consistent throughout, and are the reason why Krav Maga works well under extremely stressful conditions. They enable practitioners to assimilate higher-level threats more readily.

The Weapon

Handguns, which come in many shapes, sizes and types, appear in all scenarios presented here. For this book, there is some value in making a distinction between a semiautomatic handgun and a revolver. While revolvers still outnumber semiautomatics in the U.S., those numbers are narrowing.

It's recommended that if you're training to defend against handgun threats, you should have at least a cursory knowledge of the different types of handguns and how handguns work.

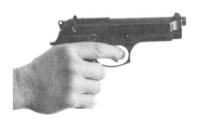

Semiautomatic handgun

A semiautomatic has a "slide" on the top of the gun that loads a round (bullet) into the chamber in preparation for the next shot. When held, the slide will not function properly, likely preventing a new round from being loaded and perhaps causing the weapon to malfunction. This is significant if the defender, once making the takeaway, chooses to use the weapon. It will be necessary to "tap and rack," or load another round by clearing the chamber.

Note: If there is already a round in the chamber, holding the slide will NOT affect that round or prevent it from firing.

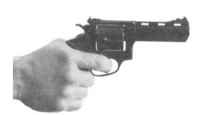

Revolver

A revolver has a cylinder, instead of a slide, that prepares the next round for firing. When held, the cylinder will not turn, preventing a new round from moving into place. This will not cause a malfunction in the revolver. Note: If the revolver is already cocked and loaded, holding the cylinder will NOT keep it from firing that round.

Important Note: NEVER train with a live (real) handgun, even if it's unloaded.

The Assailant

Handguns, when carried by criminals, are often used to intimidate, threaten, move, take property or kill. An assailant using a handgun typically derives "power" from the weapon. This is noteworthy, since once an attempted defense is made, the assailant loses this "power" and will also be in a life or death struggle. In the situations presented here, the assailant is within two to four feet (or even less) of the defender, choosing a close proximity to intimidate the defender and disguise his intentions from other parties.

Important Considerations

Critical thinking is essential when attempting to analyze a self-defense situation and determine the best course of action in the moment. When dealing with gun threats, there are many factors that go into establishing the best course of action. In order to do this in "real" time, under stress, you should commit to memory a few tangible (though not concrete) reference points that may serve to reduce reaction time.

In the handgun section, references will be made to "centerline," "live" side, "dead" side, "short" side and "long" side:

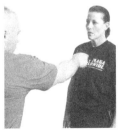

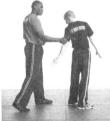

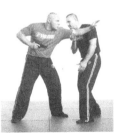

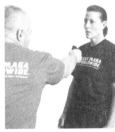

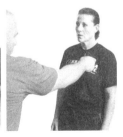

| Centerline | Movement to live side | Movement to dead side | Short side off to defender's right | Short side off to defender's left |

Centerline: the relative center of the defender's body.

Live side: the side of your body where attacks from the assailant are most readily available (generally thought of as inside the elbows or the front of the body).

Dead side: the side of your body where attacks from the assailant are least readily available (generally thought of as outside the elbows or the back of the body).

Short side: this refers to the proximity of the line of fire in relation to the centerline of the defender and the area of the body with the shortest line off the body.

Long side: this refers to the proximity of the line of fire in relation to the centerline of the defender and the area of the body with the longest line off the body.

After a disarm is made, the defender has several "after action" options available. Some of these are:

- tapping and racking the weapon (make it ready to fire), keeping the assailant in the line of fire
- using the weapon dry or cold (i.e., striking with it)
- using personal weapons/combatives
- accessing own weapon.

Regardless of which action you choose, all should serve to put you in a safer position.

Important Safety in Training Note: Do NOT put your finger on the trigger or at "ready" when training any handgun defenses as it may get broken.

EDGED WEAPONS

An edged weapon, while typically a knife, could be any short instrument used to cut or stab, such as a broken bottle, scissors, box cutter, screwdriver, etc. There are several key factors that should be considered when dealing with a threat as opposed to an attack. The behavior of the assailant is different from one who is actively stabbing or slashing at the defender. The assailant may want to gain information or property from the victim, take the victim hostage and/or move the victim to another location. Depending on the nature and context of the threat, a knife-wielding assailant has the ability to threaten the intended victim from close, intermediate and long-range distances, at various angles and heights, and by placing the edged weapon at different parts of the victim's body.

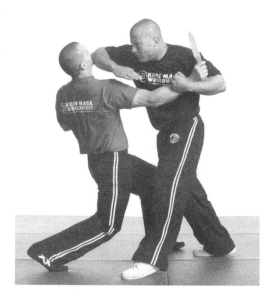

Our experiences have taught us that each passing second may allow the situation to escalate into a more dangerous and dynamic scenario, one where the assailant actively attacks with the edged weapon by stabbing and slashing repeatedly at the intended victim. Just like in basic handgun, the technical principles for addressing knife threats are Redirect, Control, Attack and Takeaway. The tactical responses generally recommended are: (1) escape, (2) use an improvised weapon or shield, and/or (3) engage with personal weapons. It's important to note that once an initial defense is made, there are four common responses from the assailant: switch knife hands, thrust the knife forward, pull the knife away, and/or strike. The techniques prescribed here are designed to address all of these concerns.

The Weapon

An edged weapon may be a dedicated weapon, such as a knife carried on one's person, or a weapon of convenience, such as scissors or broken glass. While the actual attack range is limited, the edged weapon presents multiple problems for defenders.

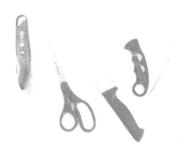

Edged weapons are easily concealed and, quite often, victims are unaware of the presence of a knife (for example). Edged weapons are typically easy to wield and difficult to isolate for the defender. Such weapons are always "live," never run out of "ammo" and almost never fail. For these reasons, among others, edged weapons are often considered the hardest to deal with. In addition, according to police reports submitted annually to the FBI, a person in the U.S. who is stabbed by a knife is 20 percent more likely to die than one who suffers a gun shot.

The Assailant

A person willing to use such a weapon is characteristically of a different mindset than those preferring other, longer-range weapons. An assailant choosing to brandish and use an edged weapon is willing to go "hands on"—to get bloody, to feel metal against bone and tendon, and to feel the life leave the victim. A person with this capacity must be met with equal or greater ferocity if the defender is to have a chance of survival.

BASIC DEFENSE PRINCIPLES

Redirect: Move the line of fire off of your body or the edge away from your body.

Control: Get control of the weapon or weapon hand.

Attack: Send aggressive counterattacks to the assailant.

Takeaway: Disarm the assailant.

Generally, the defender's hands are down by the sides. Bringing the hands up and then making a defense is a "bigger" movement that is much more obvious to the assailant. If the assailant orders the defender's hands up, this is an ideal time to make the defense (if in range), since the assailant expects movement.

HANDGUN THREATS

In order to simplify assimilation of the information, assume the handgun is being held in the right hand in all of the scenarios given.

Important Note for handgun threats from the back/side: When threatened from the dead side, it's often hard or impossible to see the weapon without first turning. In all of the defenses described, where possible, it is advised to look and see which hand holds the weapon before deciding a course of action.

BASIC GUN THREAT FROM FRONT (DEAD-SIDE OPTION)

Handgun Threats

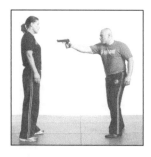

THREAT: The assailant presents the handgun at your centerline or closer to your right. In this case, it is at your chest, although it could be at your head or abdomen.

DANGER: You may be shot or taken to another location, where further crimes will be committed.

SOLUTION: The line of fire is to your centerline or towards your right, which dictates redirecting the line of fire in that direction.

1. Using the smallest move possible, bring your left hand up and place your index finger at the side of the weapon. Move the weapon in a straight line to your right, bringing your left shoulder forward to increase your reach and blading your body to make you, the target, smaller.

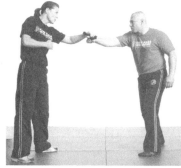

2. Grab the weapon's barrel and turn it sharply away from you, more or less parallel to the ground; begin putting your weight on the weapon as soon as possible.

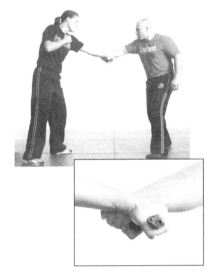

3. Leading with your left food, immediately burst forward, preferably pinning the gun against the assailant's body (at or near the stomach). Maintaining your weight on the weapon throughout, punch to the assailant's face. Note: It may be necessary to throw multiple punches, but you should keep your weight on the weapon and be prepared to continue moving forward in case the assailant is driven back as a result of the strikes.

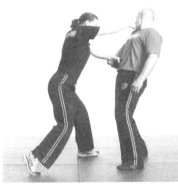

4. As you recoil your punch, keep your hand and arm close to your body. Reach under the handgun and grab the hammer and sight portion of the weapon. Break the assailant's grip on the weapon by rotating it sharply (about 90°).

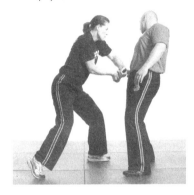

5. Pull the weapon back to your body. Do not move your feet until you have complete control of the weapon.

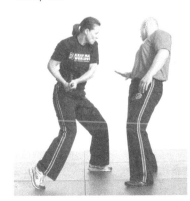

BASIC GUN THREAT FROM FRONT "CUPPING" DEFENSE (LIVE-SIDE OPTION)

Handgun Threats

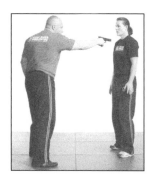

THREAT: The assailant presents the handgun at your centerline or closer to your left. In this case, it is at your chest, although it could be at your head or abdomen.

DANGER: You may be shot or taken to another location, where further crimes will be committed.

SOLUTION: The line of fire is to your centerline or towards your left, which dictates redirecting the line of fire in that direction.

1. Using the smallest move possible, bring your right hand up and place your index finger at the side of the weapon. Move the weapon in a straight line to your left, bringing your right shoulder forward to increase your reach and blading your body to make you, the target, smaller.

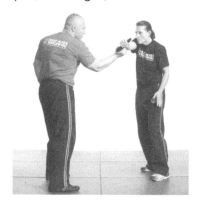

2–3. Grab the weapon's barrel and turn it sharply away from you, more or less parallel to the ground. Immediately bring your left hand up and under to the hammer portion of the weapon, building a "wall" to maintain control. Maintaining control of the weapon throughout, immediately front kick to the groin.

4. Break the assailant's grip on the weapon by turning it sharply towards him and down.

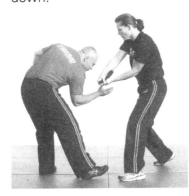

5. Pull the weapon back 5 to your body. Do not move your feet until you have complete control of the weapon.

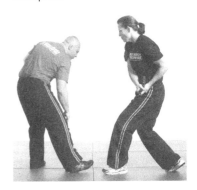

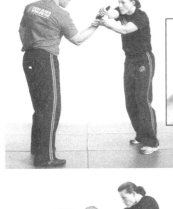

Note: It is possible to punch then make the cupping technique instead of kicking, but in most cases this is preferred because the control is stronger. It is also possible to redirect to the right and make a cupping technique, but the regular defense (dead-side option; page 338) is generally preferred.

Handgun Threats

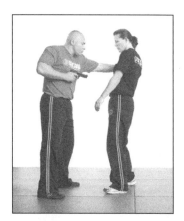

THREAT: The assailant presents the handgun at your centerline or closer to your right and uses his left hand to brace against you or push you backward. He holds the handgun back, close to his body.

DANGER: You may be shot or taken to another location, where further crimes will be committed.

SOLUTION: You determine that there is enough space between the weapon and the assailant to facilitate a redirection. The line of fire is to your centerline or towards your right, which dictates redirecting the line of fire in that direction. Because your weight is being forced back, the pushing/bracing hand must be addressed.

1. Using the smallest move possible, bring your right hand up to the hand touching you and perform a sweeping motion to clear the assailant's hand (this is similar to an outside defense, starting on page 172).

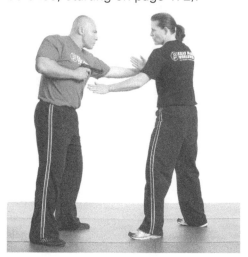

2–5. Blade your body and perform the regular gun from the front defense (dead-side option; see page 338).

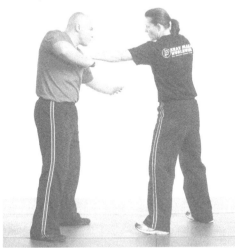

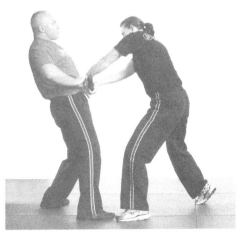

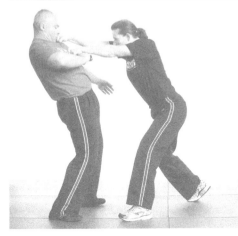

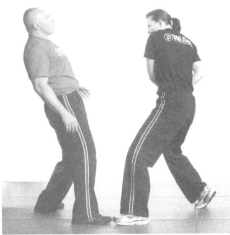

Note: It is possible that your hands are up when the threat occurs. In this case, you'll be unable to clear the hand by sweeping from the inside. The solution here is to clear the hand using a plucking motion, similar to the one used in many basic self-defense techniques. The rest of the defense would remain unchanged.

GUN THREAT WITH HAND AT CHEST (NO SPACE FOR REDIRECTION)

Handgun Threats

This defense is nearly identical to the Machine Gun Takedown on page 282.

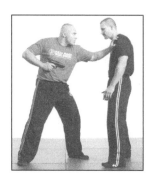

THREAT: The assailant presents the handgun and uses his left hand to brace against you or push you backward. He holds the handgun back, bracing it against his body.

DANGER: You may be shot or taken to another location, where further crimes will be committed.

SOLUTION: You determine there is not enough space between the weapon and the assailant to facilitate a redirection, and the hand bracing at your chest or even your left shoulder is forcing your weight back.

1. Using your right hand, grab the assailant's left elbow.

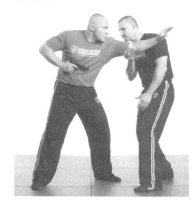

2. While lowering your body and pulling yourself forward, pull the assailant's arm towards and past your body using this grip. Stay very close to the assailant, ending up either beside or just behind him. Slide your left arm up and under the weapon arm and pin it to the assailant's body.

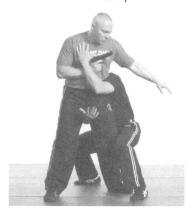

3. With the side of your head against the assailant's body, shoot your right hand up and between his legs, as if you're trying to grab his beltline.

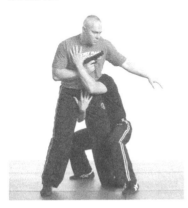

4–5. With your hips close to the assailant, lift with your legs (NOT your back) and pull your right arm back towards you. This action should cause the assailant's feet to go up and back and his head to go down towards the ground. Note: You do not need to lift the assailant very high off the ground—just a few inches. In actuality, lifting the assailant too high may allow him to spin in towards you.

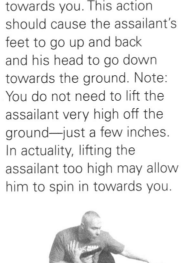

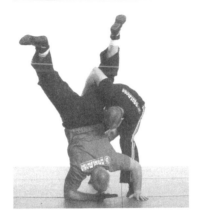

6. Drive the assailant into the ground, bringing your body down on top of him. As you do this, use elbow strikes to the back of his head. *Note:* The weapon should be under the assailant's body, but it's possible that it was dropped during the takedown and fell away from you. Take note to secure it after rendering the assailant unable to continue fighting.

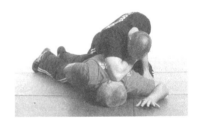

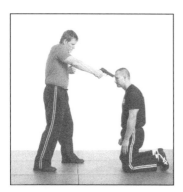

THREAT: The assailant presents the handgun while you're on your knees.

DANGER: You may be shot or taken to another location, where further crimes will be committed.

SOLUTION: In this case, the weapon is directed at your centerline. Bursting forward and counterattacking is not feasible or possible because of your body position (it simply takes too long to get up from your knees).

1–2. Perform the cupping technique by redirecting with your right hand and controlling further with your left.

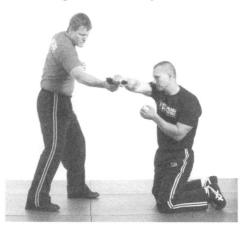

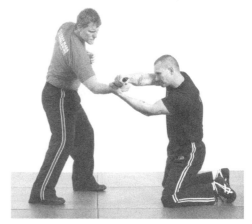

3. Once the "wall" is built, begin rising from your knees, making sure all movements are forward, towards the assailant. *Note:* It is likely the assailant will pull back on the weapon. This action will help bring you up off your knees.

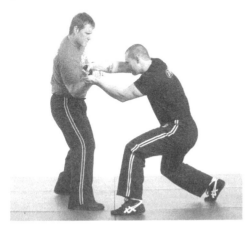

4. Redirecting the line of fire slightly upward, deliver a knee or kick to the groin. A headbutt is also a viable option, but, in this case, the line of fire should not be redirected up.

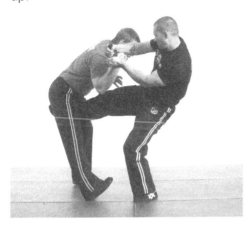

5–6. Break the assailant's grip on the weapon by rotating it sharply (about 90°) and pull the weapon back to your body. Do not move your feet until you have complete control of the weapon.

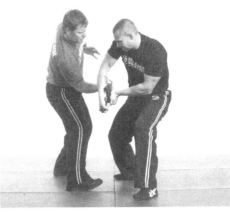

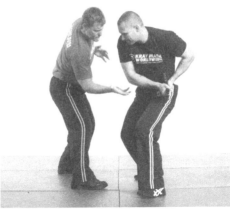

Note: This defense can be made to either direction depending on the environment and the location of the line of fire.

Handgun Threats

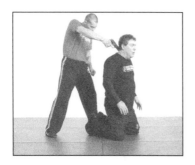

THREAT: The assailant points the handgun at the back of your head while you're on your knees.

DANGER: You may be shot or taken to another location, where further crimes will be committed.

SOLUTION: Turning and bursting to counterattack is not feasible because of your body position.

1. Bring your hands up towards the handgun, keeping them close to your body and out of sight of the assailant.

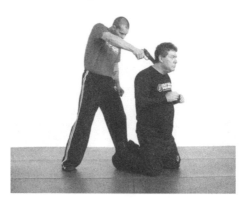

2. Using your right hand, grab the barrel and point the muzzle forward, away from you. Place your left hand at the back of the handgun, building a "wall" of control.

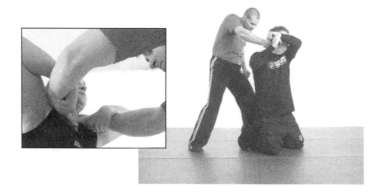

3. Immediately and sharply turn the handgun towards the right. This action will create immense pressure on the assailant's wrist, creating the disarm.

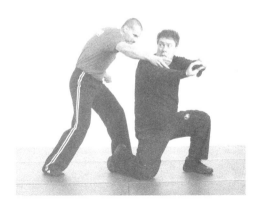

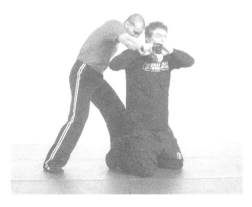

4. Extend both arms forward to completely remove the assailant's hand from the weapon.

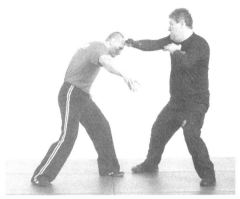

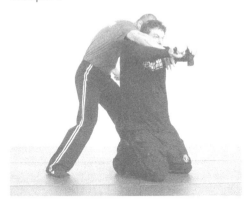

5–7. Turn and counterattack immediately with strikes to the groin before getting up to your feet for further counters and/or disengaging.

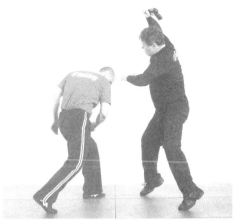

Variation: After making the takeaway, it may also be possible to shoulder roll forward and away from the assailant before turning to face him.

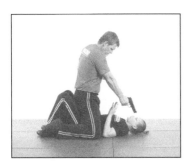

THREAT: While you're on your back, the assailant straddles you and holds the handgun to your head.

DANGER: You may be shot or taken to another location, where further crimes will be committed.

SOLUTION: There are multiple variables in this situation. You must control the weapon and make a takeaway before making a traditional counterattack. In this case, escaping the position is very important.

1. Using your right hand to redirect the weapon to the left, perform the cupping technique. Note: The redirection is important—if it's done to the other side, the assailant is likely to use the non-weapon hand to post on the ground and prevent escape.

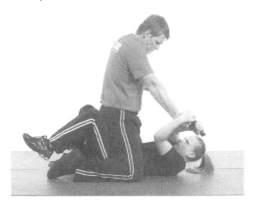

2. Take the weapon up and away from you, towards the ground, while bucking your hips up. If possible, trap the assailant's foot on the same side with your foot.

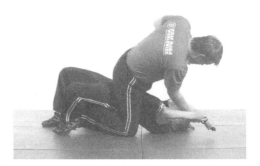

3. Buck your hips upward, towards your head and left shoulder, continuing to push the ground with your feet until you end up on top.

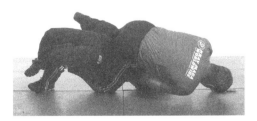

4–7. Strike with the weapon, working your way down the assailant's body to the groin, making sure to keep the line of fire away from you.

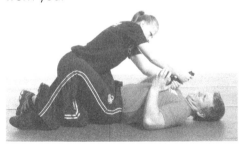

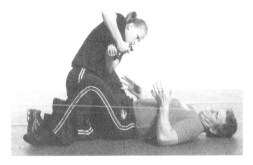

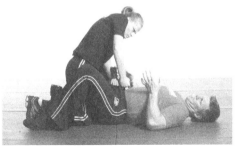

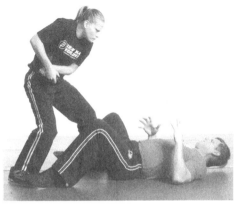

Note: You should consider your physical state in the "after action" portion of this defense. Since it's likely that a struggle put you there, it may be advisable to maneuver first to your knees then, if you feel okay, up to your feet. Otherwise, operate from your knees until you feel that you can stand without falling back down.

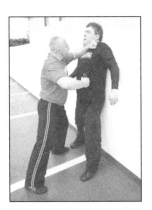

THREAT: The assailant presents the handgun to your side while using his left forearm to pin you against a wall. The short side is to your left as a result of the position the assailant is put in because of the pin.

DANGER: You may be shot or taken to another location, where further crimes will be committed.

SOLUTION: You determine there is restriction caused by the pin against the wall. The short side is to your left, which dictates redirecting the line of fire in that direction.

1. Redirect the line of fire by grabbing the barrel with your left hand and turning the muzzle to your left.

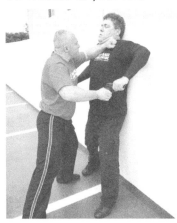

2–3. Counterattack with a strike to the head with your right hand. To make the takeaway, pull the assailant's wrist towards you and turn the muzzle sharply towards the assailant.

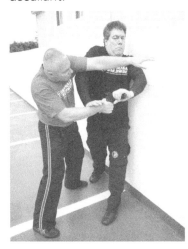

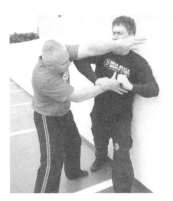

4. Counterattack with further strikes to the head, using the weapon. *Note:* When using a handgun "dry," be sure the line of fire stays away from you at all times.

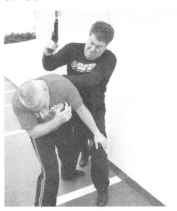

VARIATION: It's possible that the assailant uses his forearm to apply pressure lower on your chest. In this case, you may choose to redirect the assailant's forearm with your left hand.

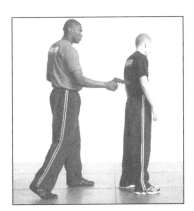

THREAT: The assailant presents the handgun, touching the weapon to your lower back. Note that the weapon could be held higher on the back or at the back of the head.

DANGER: You may be shot or taken to another location, where further crimes will be committed.

SOLUTION: The line of fire is to your centerline or towards your right, which dictates redirecting the line of fire in that direction. Remember, you must look to insure the "off hand" is not actually the weapon hand.

1. Keeping your feet in place and leading with your left arm, turn to face the assailant, redirecting the line of fire by moving the weapon with your arm and blading your body. Reaching your left hand deep under the assailant's arm, burst towards the assailant. Your left foot should be outside of the assailant's right foot.

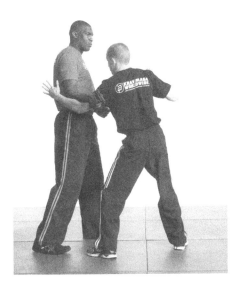

steps 2–8 continued on next page

continued from previous page

2–3. Bring your left arm up, trapping the weapon arm against your body. With your right arm, strike with an elbow to the assailant's face while sliding your left arm back to the wrist of the weapon hand. It is important that there are no gaps or spaces between your wrist, the defender's wrist or your body. Your controlling hand should be in a fist and pinned tightly to your body.

4. Counter with knees and/or kicks to the groin (additional upper body combatives are also possible).

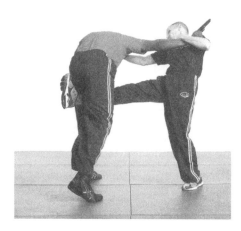

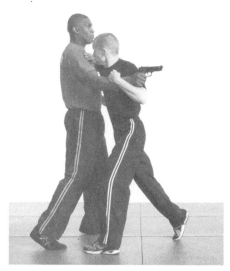

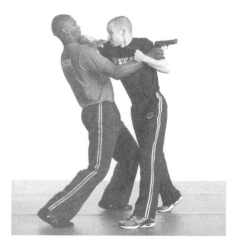

5. Bringing your left shoulder slightly forward, reach over with your right hand, pinky side up, and grab the barrel of the weapon. Keep your eyes on the assailant and be sure not to turn your back.

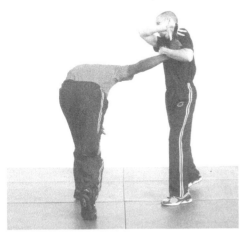

6. To break the grip, snap the muzzle of the weapon down towards the ground, bringing your entire arm down.

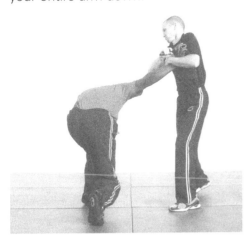

7. Lift the weapon straight up for the takeaway.

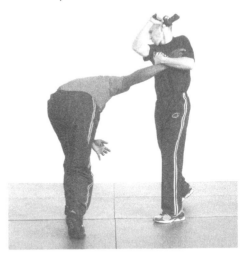

8. Deliver counterattacks, such as elbows and/or weapon strikes, and get out.

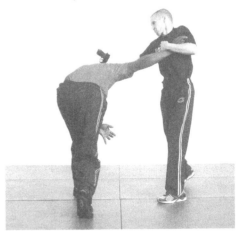

GUN THREAT, HOSTAGE POSITION

Handgun Threats

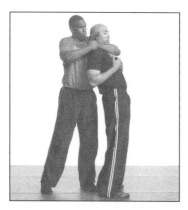

THREAT: The assailant stands with his chest to your back. He loops his left arm around the front of your throat and points the handgun at the side of your head.

DANGER: You may be shot or taken to another location, where further crimes will be committed.

SOLUTION: Because the assailant is to your dead side and is controlling at least a portion of your body, the redirection and takeaway are made before the counterattack.

1. Bring your hands up towards the handgun, keeping them close to your body and out of sight of the assailant.

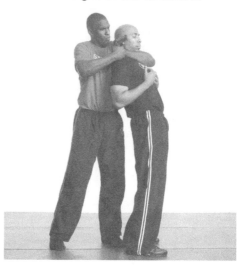

2. Using your right hand, grab the barrel and redirect the muzzle forward (this turn should be about 90°).

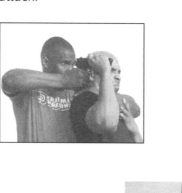

3–4. Place your left hand at the back of the handgun, building a "wall" of control.

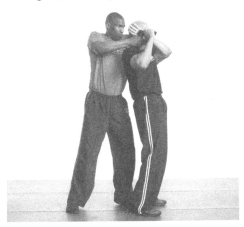

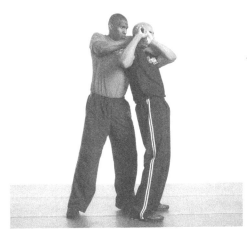

5. Push the handgun forward. Immediately and sharply turn the handgun towards the right. This action will create immense pressure on the assailant's wrist, creating the disarm. While shooting your hips back to further separate the assailant from the weapon, extend both arms forward to completely remove the assailant's hand from the weapon.

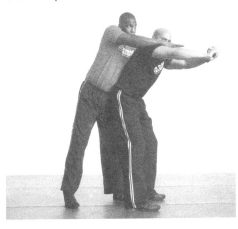

6. Turn and counterattack immediately before moving to a safe distance.

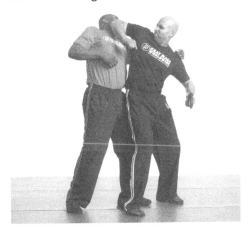

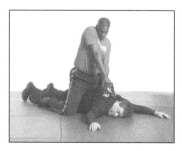

THREAT: The assailant straddles you while you lie face-down on the ground. He holds the handgun at the back of your head.

DANGER: You may be shot or taken to another location, where further crimes will be committed.

SOLUTION: There are multiple variables in this situation. You must control the weapon and make a takeaway before making a traditional counterattack. In this case, escaping the position is very important.

1. Bring your hands up towards your head, keeping them close to the ground.

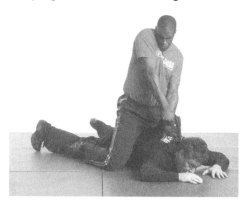

2. Using your right hand (assuming your face is turned to the right), grab the barrel and redirect the weapon forward and slightly to the right. The muzzle should be angled away from your face. Note: The angle of redirection/placement is important. If the initial round is discharged, any debris should go away from your face, not towards it.

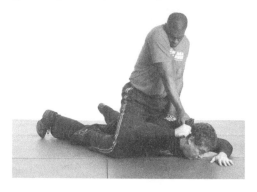

3. With your left hand, control the wrist of the weapon hand while lifting your upper body.

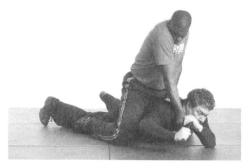

4. With your right shoulder at or near the assailant's elbow, drive that shoulder forward and pull the gun back, under your body.

5–6. As the assailant goes over your head, take your body back and under the assailant.

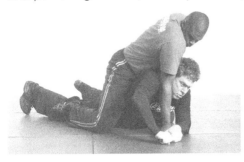

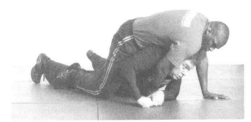

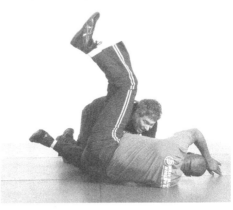

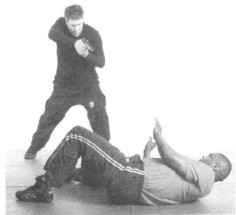

Note: You should consider your physical state in the "after action" portion of this defense. Since it's likely that a struggle put you there, it may be advisable to maneuver first to your knees then, if you feel okay, up to your feet. Otherwise, operate from your knees until you feel that you can stand without falling back down.

EDGED-WEAPON THREATS

In order to simplify assimilation of the information, assume the knife is being held in the right hand in all of the scenarios given. The emphasis is almost always on controlling the weapon and counterattacking aggressively. While disarms are shown, the "real" defense is in the offense. Counterattacks should be of a nature that renders the assailant unable or unwilling to continue the attack.

EDGED WEAPON TOUCHING OR AT SHORT DISTANCE OFF THE BODY

Edged-Weapon Threats

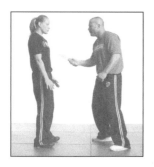

THREAT: The assailant is close to you and presents the knife to the front of your body.

DANGER: The knife may be touching you or simply held close to your body. The knife is not necessarily held statically—the assailant may be moving it around, giving directions, pointing, threatening, etc. The assailant may wish to move you to another location.

SOLUTION: Because of the proximity of the threat, you should attempt to control the weapon hand and counterattack aggressively.

1. With your left hand, grab the assailant's weapon-hand wrist, redirecting the weapon towards your right side.

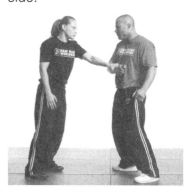

2–3. As soon as possible, reach your right hand to control the weapon hand, covering the hand as much as possible. Extend your arms away from you, applying weight and creating distance. Tuck your chin behind your right shoulder to minimize the chance of being struck in the face.

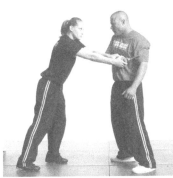

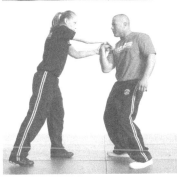

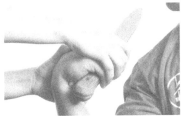

4. As soon as you attain control, send a front kick to the groin. (If the assailant's body is angled, a round kick to the groin, using the ball of your foot, may be more applicable.) After the initial counterattack, follow with additional counters, maintaining control of the weapon hand and keeping the weapon away from your body. Kicks to the groin and face (if the assailant is doubled over) are preferable.

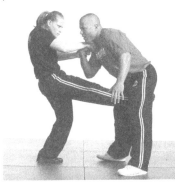

5. Maintain control at the wrist using your whole body, with the palm of your right hand applying pressure to the knuckles of the assailant's weapon hand. The pressure should force the fingers surrounding the knife to open. While maintaining contact, scrape

the weapon out of the assailant's hand.

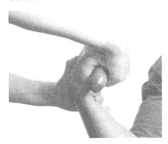

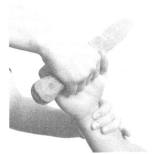

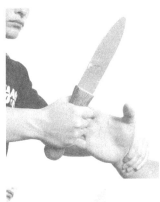

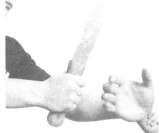

Edged-Weapon Threats

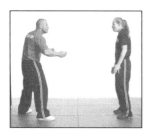

THREAT: The assailant stands further away from you and presents the knife to the front of your body.

DANGER: The threat may be the same as with the knife closer to the body but, because of the distance, getting the second hand on quickly is difficult to do. The knife is not necessarily held statically—the assailant may be moving it around, giving directions, pointing, threatening, etc.

SOLUTION: Because of the distance, instead of controlling the weapon hand, you should emphasize redirecting the weapon, counterattacking, and escaping or attaining an object that may be used as a weapon or shield.

1–2. Using the palm of your left hand, redirect the weapon hand towards your right with a quick, explosive striking movement to the back of the assailant's hand. Note: The redirection is slightly up, which yields less resistance. Your left shoulder should move forward, which angles your body and increases your reach.

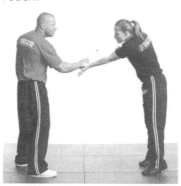

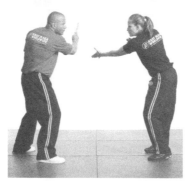

3. Immediately after redirecting the weapon hand, advance with a front kick to the groin, moving at an angle in the opposite direction of the redirected weapon hand. Immediately seek to escape or acquire an object that may be used as a shield or weapon.

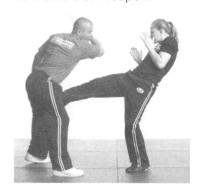

Edged-Weapon Threats

[THREAT: This close-range situation has the weapon likely touching the right side of your neck.

DANGER: Here, due to the proximity to the carotid artery, only a small movement by the assailant is required to inflict severe injury or death.

SOLUTION: It becomes necessary to recognize the "open" area. In other words, you must analyze the orientation of the weapon as it relates to the direction needed to inflict harm and redirect the weapon in the opposite direction.

1. Using your left hand, grab the weapon hand at the wrist, redirecting it away from your neck, while moving your head in the opposite direction (dead side).

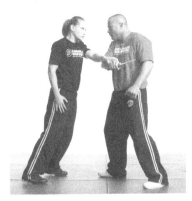

2. Bring your right hand up immediately to cover the weapon hand of the assailant, extending your arms to create space and leverage on the wrist. Note: Rotate your redirecting hand so that your palm faces in the direction of the assailant. This action helps facilitate getting the second hand on and offers the palm, as opposed to just the thumb, as a "backstop."

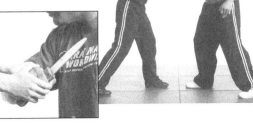

steps 3–4 continued on next page

continued from previous page

3. Immediately after gaining control of the weapon hand, send a front kick to the groin. Send multiple counters, maintaining control of the weapon hand and keeping the weapon away from your body. Kicks to the groin and face (if the assailant is doubled over) are preferable.

4. Maintain control at the wrist using your whole body, with the palm of your right hand applying pressure to the knuckles of the assailant's weapon hand. The pressure should force the fingers surrounding the knife to open. While maintaining contact, scrape the weapon out of the assailant's hand.

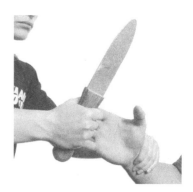

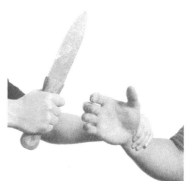

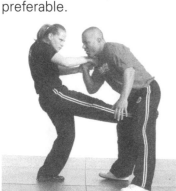

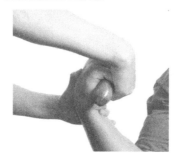

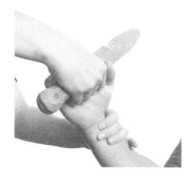

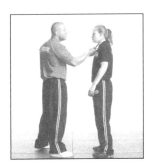

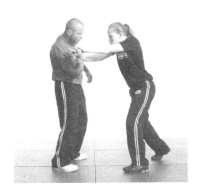

1. Using your right hand, grab the weapon hand at the wrist, redirecting it away from your neck, while moving your head in the opposite direction (live side).

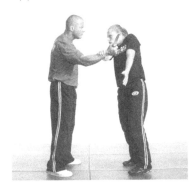

THREAT: This close-range situation has the weapon likely touching the left side of your neck.

DANGER: Here, due to the proximity to the carotid artery, only a small movement by the assailant is required to inflict severe injury or death.

SOLUTION: It becomes necessary to recognize the "open" area. In other words, you must analyze the orientation of the weapon as it relates to the direction needed to inflict harm and redirect the weapon in the opposite direction.

2. With your left hand, immediately cover the assailant's weapon hand and straighten your arms to create space and pressure. Immediately counterattack with a front kick to the groin.

3. Transition both thumbs to the back of the assailant's weapon hand (at the knuckle line) while maintaining pressure on the wrist (Cavalier #3, as shown on page 258).

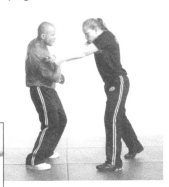

steps 4–6 continued on next page

continued from previous page

4. Maintaining weight and pressure on the assailant's wrist, move your right hand to cover the assailant's weapon hand and continue to control the assailant's wrist with your left hand (Cavalier #1, as shown on page 256).

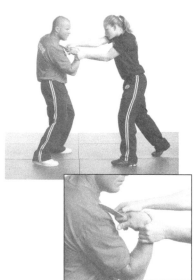

5. If necessary or possible, send another kick to the groin, maintaining the wrist control.

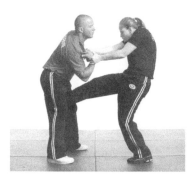

6. Using your whole body, maintain control at the wrist, with the palm of your right hand applying pressure to the knuckles of the assailant's weapon hand. The pressure should force the fingers surrounding the knife to open. While maintaining contact, scrape the weapon out of the assailant's hand.

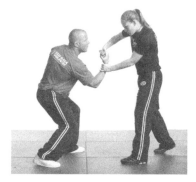

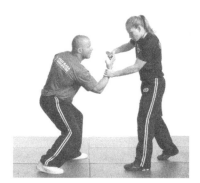

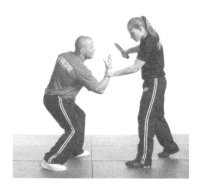

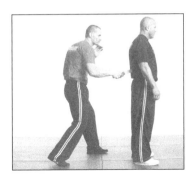

THREAT: The assailant touches the knife to your back.

DANGER: While the assailant's intent may be to move you or take property, you are very vulnerable to stabs to the back.

SOLUTION: When responding to this threat, it's important to take a quick look over or around your shoulder to determine that the weapon (not the assailant's hand or fingers) is actually at your back and not held in his back hand. Krav Maga practitioners familiar with basic handgun defenses will find the response to this threat very similar.

1. After determining that the weapon is indeed placed at your back, turn towards the left, with your left arm leading the motion.

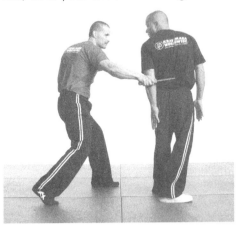

2. As your left arm redirects the weapon, continue to reach with your left and burst in very deep, reaching your left arm towards the assailant's underarm. Be sure to push the weapon out and away from your body.

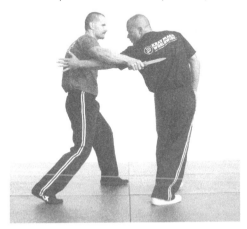

steps 3–8 continued on next page

continued from previous page

3. Bring your left arm up, trapping the assailant's arm to your body. Your arm should slide to the assailant's wrist while delivering an elbow to the assailant's face with your right arm.

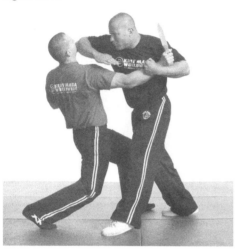

4. Follow the elbow with multiple counterattacks, including knees, kicks, etc.

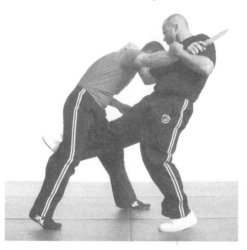

5. Maintaining control and leverage on the wrist, reach over with your right hand and cover the weapon hand.

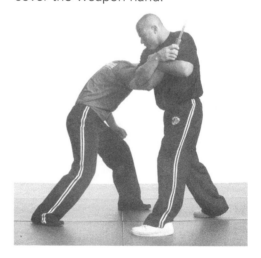

6. While applying pressure to the assailant's wrist and shoulder, rotate the weapon hand so that the palm faces up and his fingers are forced open.

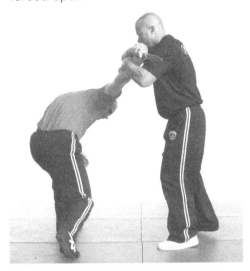

7. Without losing contact or control, scrape the knife out of the assailant's hand.

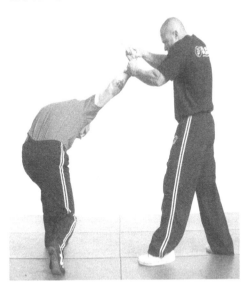

Edged-Weapon Threats

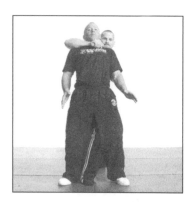

1. Bring your hands up, keeping them close to your body and concealed from the assailant's sight.

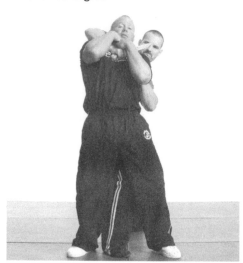

THREAT: The assailant drapes his weapon arm over your shoulder and places the knife against your throat or neck. Often, you will be pulled backward, compromising balance.

DANGER: While the assailant's intent may be to move you or take property, and/or give demands to third parties, you are very vulnerable. With this threat, due to the proximity to the carotid artery and/or throat, only a small movement by the assailant is required to inflict severe injury or death.

SOLUTION: Redirect and control the weapon hand while turning to face the assailant and counterattacking. Krav Maga practitioners familiar with basic headlock defenses will find commonality with aspects of this defense.

2. Reaching first with your right hand, pluck at the assailant's wrist, redirecting the weapon hand down and away from your neck while immediately adding your left hand for better control. Tuck your chin.

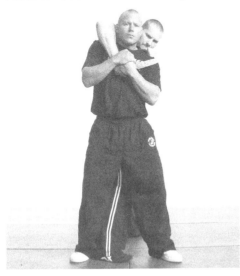

3. Raise your right shoulder to create additional space and leverage.

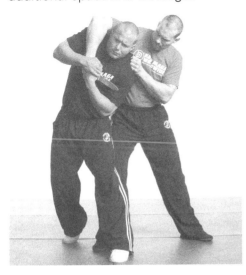

4. Step out and around the assailant with your left leg. Your head and neck should be tight against the back of the assailant's forearm and triceps area—no space!

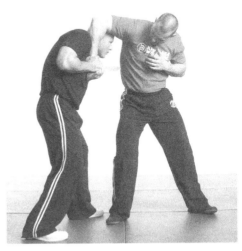

5. Transition your left hand to cover the weapon hand and control his wrist with your right hand. Stab with your entire body by advancing toward the assailant.

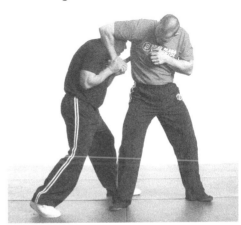

INDEX

ABOUT THE CONTRIBUTORS

Darren Levine, a 6th-degree black belt, is the founder of the nonprofit Krav Maga Association and serves as the Chief Executive Officer and U.S. Chief Instructor of Krav Maga Worldwide. He has trained thousands of civilians and hundreds of law enforcement and military personnel around the world. In addition, Darren is a Deputy District Attorney who has won the California Deputy District Attorney of the Year Award. Darren has lectured widely on use-of-force issues and is well-known in the law enforcement community. In the Los Angeles District Attorney's office, he serves as a senior member of the Crimes Against Peace Officers Section (CAPOS), an elite unit that prosecutes offenders who murder, or attempt to murder, police officers. In his dual roles as Krav Maga Chief Instructor and as a Deputy District Attorney, he has dedicated his life to the safety of others.

John Whitman is a 4th-degree black belt in Krav Maga and the president of Krav Maga Worldwide. He holds instructor's diplomas from both the Krav Maga Association of America and Wingate University in Israel, and has trained at the Israeli Military Institute in personal protection and installation protection. John has been teaching Krav Maga since 1994, and has trained thousands of civilians as well as law enforcement and military units, including the Air Force Office of Special Investigations Antiterrorist Specialty Team and the Special Operations Group for the Japanese Self-Defense Force. John has also published a number of books, including several 24 novels.

Bas Rutten, the author of the foreword, is a Dutch mixed martial arts fighter who is the former Ultimate Fighting Championship (UFC) Heavyweight Champion and a three-time King of Pancrase. He is a certified MTBN Thai Boxing instructor and a Pancrase instructor. He is also a 5th-degree black belt in Kyokushin karate and a 2nd-degree black belt in Tae Kwon Do. He founded The Bas Rutten System and has written several martial art books and made instructional videos. Bas has been the color commentator for the Pride Fighting Championships in Japan, and is currently the spokesperson for the International Fight League (IFL). He is considered by many to be the best Dutch fighter in mixed martial arts history.